Yoga

FOR

DUMMIES®

PORTABLE EDITION

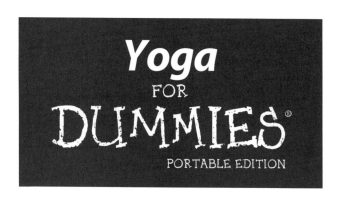

Yoga
FOR
DUMMIES®
PORTABLE EDITION

**by Georg Feuerstein, PhD,
and Larry Payne, PhD**

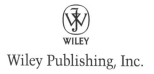

Wiley Publishing, Inc.

Yoga For Dummies®, Portable Edition

Published by
Wiley Publishing, Inc.
111 River St.
Hoboken, NJ 07030-5774
www.wiley.com

For general information on our other products and services, please contact our Customer Care Department within the U.S. at 877-762-2974, outside the U.S. at 317-572-3993, or fax 317-572-4002.

For technical support, please visit www.wiley.com/techsupport.

Wiley also publishes its books in a variety of electronic formats. Some content that appears in print may not be available in electronic books.

ISBN: 978-0-470-59193-2

Manufactured in the United States of America

10 9 8 7 6 5 4 3 2 1

Publisher's Acknowledgments

Editor: Elizabeth Kuball

Composition Services: Indianapolis Composition Services Department

Special Photography: Blaine Michioka/Rainbow Photography

Cover Photo: © iStock

WILEY

Table of Contents

Introduction

● ●

*M*ore than six million Americans practice Yoga of one kind or another, and more or less regularly. Many more millions of Yoga practitioners live in other parts of the world. They aren't all dummies, and neither are you, really. The fact that you're reading *Yoga For Dummies* proves that curiosity is alive and kicking in you and that you're willing to learn. In our definition, a dummy is not someone who is abysmally ignorant and stupid, but someone who knows that he or she doesn't know something and actively seeks to fill this gap with the best knowledge available. Someone like you.

About This Book

Perhaps *Yoga For Dummies* is the first book on Yoga you have ever held in your hands. In this case, you're starting at the right place. More likely, however, you've leafed through quite a few other books (there is definitely no shortage of publications dealing with Yoga exercises). Not all those publications are either sound or helpful. Why, then, should you take this book seriously? We have a two-part answer for you.

First, the information you find in *Yoga For Dummies* is based on our extensive study and practice of Yoga. Between us, we have 55 years of experience with Yoga. One author (Georg Feuerstein) is internationally recognized as a leading expert on the Yoga tradition and has authored many seminal works on it. The other author (Larry Payne) has a thriving practice as a Yoga teacher in Los Angeles, where he teaches and responds to his clients' specific health challenges, notably back problems, and is featured in popular Yoga and back videos. In this book, we merge our respective areas of expertise to create a reliable and user-friendly introductory book that can also serve you as a beginner's reference work on an ongoing basis.

Second, we are both dedicated to motivating you to practice this system, which we have seen work minor and major miracles. We've committed our lives to making Yoga available to anyone who cares about the health and wholeness of his body and mind. In short, you're in the best of hands.

Yoga For Dummies guides you slowly, step by step, into the treasure house of Yoga. And it is a fabulous treasure house! You'll find out how to unlock your body's extraordinary potential and enlist your mind to do so, and in the process strengthen your mind as well. Remember the old Latin saying, _Mens sana in corpore sane_ (A sound mind in a sound body). We show you how to improve or regain the health and wholeness of your body and mind.

Whether you're interested in becoming more flexible, fitter, less stressed out, or more peaceful and joyful, this book contains all the good counsel and practical exercises to start you in the right direction. Our presentation is based on the rich heritage of Yoga, which is the oldest system of total well-being in the world.

Thus, _Yoga For Dummies_ contains enough information to be useful also to those who have taken the first few steps into the world of Yoga and want to know about coming attractions. Above all, we've endeavored to make this book relevant to busy people like yourself. And if, after reading this guide, you become more serious about studying and practicing Yoga, consider taking a Yoga class with a qualified instructor. This book is a great guide, but nothing compares to hands-on teaching.

Yoga is not a fad. It has been around in this country for over a hundred years and has a history of approximately five millennia. It is clearly here to stay. Yoga has brought health and peace of mind to millions of people. It can do the same for you.

Icons Used in This Book

Throughout this book you'll notice little pictures in the margins. We call them *icons.* Here's what they stand for:

This icon points you toward helpful information that can make your yogic journey a little smoother. Be sure to read these morsels!

This icon flags danger ahead. Be sure to check out the information marked by this icon; you'll be glad you did!

This icon marks nerdy technical stuff that's interesting to know but probably not necessary to your understanding of Yoga. Read this and impress your friends at your next dinner party.

Sometimes the terms used in association with Yoga can be fairly jargony and strange-sounding to most people. This icon flags such words so you can pay special attention to them. If you're not careful, you may start sounding like a pro!

This icon leads you to the various routines, exercises, and postures scattered throughout the book. If it's exercises you want, keep your eyes peeled for this icon.

This icon sits next to text that cuts through the myth and mystery to expose the truth about Yoga. This is interesting stuff!

Look for this icon to find out some personal experiences we've encountered during our 55 combined years in the world of Yoga. You'll laugh, you'll cry, and you may even learn something!

Where to Go from Here

You've got your Portable Edition of *Yoga For Dummies* — now what? This portable guide is a reference, so if you need information on relaxation, head to Chapter 3. Or if you're interested in finding a beginner Yoga routine, go straight to Chapter 5. Or heck, start with Chapter 1 and read the chapters in order . . . you rebel. If you want even more advice on Yoga, from sharing Yoga with your kids to creating your own Yoga routine, check out the full-size version of *Yoga For Dummies* — simply head to your local book seller or go to www.dummies.com!

Chapter 1

Yoga 101: What You Need to Know

*T*wo or three decades ago, some people still occasionally confused *Yoga* with *yogurt.* Today, Yoga is a household word.

The fact that just about everyone has heard the word *Yoga,* however, doesn't mean that everyone knows exactly what it means. Many misconceptions still exist, even among those who practice Yoga. In this chapter, we clear up the confusion and explain what Yoga really is and how it relates to your health and happiness. We also help you see that Yoga, with its many different branches and approaches, really does offer something for everyone.

Headed to the capital

In English, you customarily write *yoga* in lowercase letters. However, throughout this book, we write the word with an initial capital letter — *Yoga* — to emphasize that Yoga is a self-contained system or tradition, like Zen, Taoism, or Hinduism. The adjective form of *Yoga* is *yogic*, which you encounter frequently in this book.

Whatever your age, weight, flexibility, or beliefs may be, you can practice and benefit from Yoga. Although it originated in India, Yoga is for all of humanity.

Understanding the True Character of Yoga

 Whenever you're told that Yoga is *just* this or *just* that, your nonsense alert should kick into action. Yoga is too comprehensive to reduce to any one thing. Yoga is like a skyscraper with many floors and numerous rooms at each level. Here's what Yoga is not:

- ✔ Yoga is not *just* gymnastics.

- ✔ Yoga is not *just* fitness training.

- ✔ Yoga is not *just* a way to control your weight.

- ✔ Yoga is not *just* a technique for stress reduction.

- ✔ Yoga is not *just* meditation.

- ✔ Yoga is not *just* the "huffing and puffing" of proper breath control.

✔ Yoga is not *just* a way to improve and maintain your health.

✔ Yoga is not *just* a spiritual tradition from India.

To put it simply, Yoga is all these things — the catch is that it's also a great deal more. (You would expect as much from a tradition that's been around for 5,000 years.) Yoga includes physical exercises that look like gymnastics — some of which have even been incorporated into Western gymnastics. These exercises help you become or stay fit and trim, control your weight, and reduce your stress level. Yoga also offers a whole range of meditation practices, including breathing techniques that exercise your lungs and calm your nervous system or charge your brain and the rest of your body with delicious energy.

Moreover, you can use Yoga as an efficient system of healthcare, one that has proven its usefulness in both restoring and maintaining health. Yoga continues to gain acceptance within the medical establishment. More and more physicians are recommending Yoga to their patients, not only for stress reduction but also as a safe and sane method of exercise, as well as physical therapy (notably, for the back and knees).

But Yoga is more than even a system of preventive or restorative healthcare. Yoga looks at health from a broad, holistic perspective that's only now being rediscovered by avant-garde medicine. This perspective appreciates the enormous influence of the mind — your psychological attitudes — on physical health.

Finding meaning: The word Yoga

 The word *Yoga* comes from the ancient *Sanskrit* language spoken by the traditional religious elite of India, the *Brahmins*. Yoga means "union" or "integration" and "discipline," so the system of Yoga is called a *unitive* or *integrating discipline*.

Yoga seeks unity at various levels. First, Yoga seeks to unite your body and mind. All too often, people separate their minds from their bodies. Some people are chronically "out of the body." They can't feel their feet or the ground beneath them, as if they hover like ghosts just above their bodies. They're unable to cope with the ordinary pressures of daily life and collapse under stress. Often, they're confused and don't understand their own emotions. They're afraid of life and easily hurt.

Many people suffer from slighter forms of this syndrome, which can make facing life squarely and mindfully a difficult task. Because they are not fully "in" the body, they tend to also be somewhat disconnected from the world around them. This causes them to daydream and avoid, rather than face, life's challenges. Through Yoga, they can reconnect their mind and emotions to the body, enabling them to live life more fully and with enjoyment.

A second problem that Yoga tackles is the split between the rational mind and the emotions. All too often, people bottle up their emotions and don't express their real feelings, choosing instead to rationalize these feelings away. If done chronically, this avoidance can become a serious health hazard. Sometimes people aren't even aware that they're suppressing their feelings — especially anger. Then anger or frustration consumes them from the inside out.

Here's how Yoga can help you with your personal growth:

- Yoga can put you in touch with your real feelings and balance your emotional life.

- Yoga can help you become less fragmented inwardly and more whole and real. In other words, it can help you understand and accept yourself and feel comfortable with who you are.

You won't have to "fake it" or reduce your life to constant role playing.

✔ Yoga can greatly improve your "hook-up" to other people. That is, you become more able to empathize and communicate with others.

Yoga is a powerful means of psychological integration. It makes you aware that you're part of a larger whole, not merely an island unto yourself. Humans can't thrive in isolation. Even the most independent individual is greatly indebted to others. When your mind and body are happily reunited, this union with others comes about naturally. The moral principles of Yoga are all embracing, encouraging you to seek kinship with everyone and everything.

Finding yourself: Are you a yogi (or yogini)?

Someone who's dedicated to the discipline of balancing mind and body through Yoga is traditionally called a *yogi* (if male) or a *yogini* (if female). In this book, we use both terms at random. Alternatively, we also use the English term *Yoga practitioner.*

A yogi or yogini who has really mastered Yoga is called a *Yoga master* or an *adept.* If such an adept also teaches (and not all of them do), he or she traditionally is called a *guru.* The Sanskrit word *guru* means literally "weighty one." According to traditional esoteric sources, the syllable *gu* signifies spiritual darkness and *ru* signifies the act of removing. Thus, a *guru* is a teacher who leads the student from darkness to light.

Very few Westerners have achieved complete mastery of Yoga, mainly because Yoga is still a relatively young movement in the West. However, at the level at which Yoga is generally taught outside its Indian homeland, many competent Yoga teachers or instructors can lend a helping hand to beginners. In this book, we hope to do just that for you.

Considering Your Options: The Eight Main Branches of Yoga

When you take a bird's-eye view of the Yoga tradition, you see a dozen major strands of development, each with its own subdivisions. Picture Yoga as a giant tree with eight branches — each branch has its own unique character, but each is also part of the same tree.

In the following sections, we cover each of these eight branches.

Bhakti Yoga: The Yoga of devotion

Bhakti Yoga (pronounced *bhuk-tee*) practitioners believe that a supreme being transcends their lives, and they feel moved to connect or even completely merge with that supreme being through acts of devotion. Bhakti Yoga includes such practices as making flower offerings, singing hymns of praise, and thinking about the divine being.

Guru Yoga: The Yoga of dedication to a master

In Guru Yoga (pronounced *goo-roo*), one's teacher is the main focus of spiritual practice. Such a teacher is expected to be enlightened or at least close to being enlightened. In Guru Yoga, you're asked to honor and meditate on your guru until you merge with him or her. Because the guru is thought to be one with the ultimate reality, this merger is believed to duplicate his or her spiritual realization in you.

Hatha Yoga: The Yoga of physical discipline

All branches of Yoga seek to achieve the same final goal, enlightenment, but Hatha Yoga (pronounced *haht-ha*) approaches this goal through the body rather than through the mind or through the emotions. Hatha Yoga practitioners believe that unless the body is properly purified and prepared, the higher stages of concentration, meditation, and ecstasy are virtually impossible to achieve — such an attempt would be like trying to climb Mount Everest without the necessary gear. Much of this book focuses on this branch of Yoga.

The body is a precious possession. Yoga asks you to take proper care of it, so that you can enjoy not only health but also longevity and, ultimately, enlightenment.

In this book, we focus on Hatha Yoga, the most popular branch of Yoga, but we avoid the common mistake of reducing it to mere physical-fitness training. Thus, we also talk about meditation and the spiritual aspects of Yoga.

Jnana Yoga: The Yoga of wisdom

Jnana Yoga (pronounced *gyah-nah*) teaches the ideal of *nondualism* — that reality is singular and your perception of countless distinct phenomena is a basic misconception. What about the chair or sofa that you're sitting on? Isn't that real? What about the light that strikes your retina? Isn't that real? Jnana Yoga masters answer these questions by saying that all these things are real at your present level of consciousness, but they aren't ultimately real as separate or distinct things. Upon enlightenment, everything melts into one, and you become one with the immortal spirit.

Feeling enlightened

To get a sense of the nature of enlightenment, sit in a warm room as still as possible, with your hands in your lap. Now sense your skin all over, which is your body's boundary separating you from the air surrounding you. As you become more aware of your body's sensations, pay special attention to the connection between your skin and the air. After a while, you'll realize that there is really no sharp boundary between your skin and the "outside" air. In your imagination, you can extend yourself further and further beyond your skin into the surrounding space. Where do you end, and where does the space begin? This experience can give you a sense of the all-comprising expansiveness of enlightenment, which knows no boundaries.

Karma Yoga: The Yoga of self-transcending action

Karma Yoga (pronounced *kahr-mah*) seeks to influence destiny positively. This path's most important principle is to act unselfishly, without attachment, and with integrity. Karma Yoga practitioners believe that all actions — whether physical, vocal, or mental — have far-reaching consequences for which we must assume full responsibility.

Mantra Yoga: The Yoga of potent sound

Mantra Yoga (pronounced *mahn-trah*) makes use of sound to harmonize the body and focus the mind. It works with a *mantra,* which can be a syllable, word, or phrase. Traditionally, practitioners receive a *mantra* from their teacher in the context of a formal initiation. They're asked to repeat it as often as possible and to keep it secret.

Good karma, bad karma, no karma

The Sanskrit term *karma* means literally "action." It stands for activity in general but also for the "invisible action" of destiny. According to Yoga, every action of body, speech, and mind produces visible and also hidden consequences. Sometimes the hidden consequences — destiny — are far more significant than the obvious repercussions.

Don't think of karma as blind destiny. You are always free to make choices. The purpose of Karma Yoga is to regulate how you act in the world so that you cease to be bound by karma. The practitioners of Karma Yoga seek not only to prevent bad karma but also to go beyond good karma to no karma at all. According to this Yoga branch, all karma binds you to the state of unenlightenment. This state is undesirable because, in it, you are neither free nor blissful.

Many Western teachers feel that initiation is not necessary and that any sound will do. You can even pick a word from the dictionary — such as *love, peace,* or *happiness.*

Raja Yoga: The Royal Yoga

Raja Yoga (pronounced *rah-jah*) means literally "Royal Yoga" and is also known as *Classical Yoga.*

When you mingle with Yoga students long enough, you can expect to hear them refer to the *eightfold path,* as codified in the *Yoga-Sutra* of Patanjali. This is the standard work of Raja Yoga. Another name for this yogic tradition is *ashtanga-yoga* (pronounced *ahsh-tahng-gah*), the "eight-limbed Yoga" — from *ashta* ("eight") and *anga* ("limb").

The sacred syllable OM

The best-known traditional mantra, used by Hindus and Buddhists alike, is the sacred syllable *om* (pronounced *ohmmm*). It's said to be the symbol of the absolute reality, the Self or spirit. It's composed of the letters *a, u, m,* and the nasal humming of the letter *m. A* corresponds to the waking state; *u* corresponds to the dream state; *m* corresponds to the state of deep sleep; and the nasal humming sound represents the ultimate reality.

The eight limbs of this prominent approach, which are designed to lead to enlightenment, or liberation, are as follows:

- ✔ *Yama* **(pronounced *yah-mah*):** Moral discipline, consisting of the practices of nonharming, truthfulness, nonstealing, chastity, and greedlessness.

- ✔ *Niyama* **(pronounced *nee-yah-mah*):** Self-restraint, consisting of the five practices of purity, contentment, austerity, self-study, and devotion to a higher principle.

- ✔ *Asana* **(pronounced *ah-sah-nah*):** Posture, which serves two basic purposes — meditation and health.

- ✔ *Pranayama* **(pronounced *prah-nah-yah-mah*):** Breath control, which raises and balances your psychosomatic energy, thus boosting your health and mental concentration.

- ✔ *Pratyahara* **(pronounced *prah-tyah-hah-rah*):** Sensory inhibition, which internalizes your consciousness to prepare the mind for the various stages of meditation.

✔ *Dharana* (pronounced *dhah-rah-nah*):
Concentration, or extended mental focusing,
which is fundamental to yogic meditation.

✔ *Dhyana* (pronounced *dhee-yah-nah*):
Meditation, the principal practice of higher
Yoga.

✔ *Samadhi* (pronounced *sah-mah-dhee*):
Ecstasy, or the experience of unitive consciousness, in which you become inwardly one with
the object of your contemplation.

Tantra Yoga: The Yoga of continuity

Tantra Yoga (pronounced *tahn-trah*) is the most complex and most widely misunderstood branch of Yoga.
In the West and in India, Tantra Yoga is often confused with "spiritualized" sex. Although sexual rituals
are used in some schools of Tantra Yoga, this isn't a
regular practice in the majority of schools. Tantra
Yoga is actually a strict spiritual discipline involving
fairly complex rituals and detailed visualizations of
deities. These deities are either visions of the divine
or the equivalent of Christianity's angels and are
invoked to aid the yogic process of contemplation.

Another name for Tantra Yoga is Kundalini Yoga
(pronounced *koon-dah-lee-nee*). The latter name,
which means "she who is coiled," hints at the
secret "serpent power" that Tantra Yoga seeks to
activate: the latent spiritual energy stored in the
human body. If you're curious about this aspect of
Yoga, you may want to read *Living with Kundalini:
The Autobiography of Gopi Krishna,* edited by
Leslie Shepard (Shambhala Publications).

Finding Your Niche: Five Basic Approaches to Yoga

Since the late 19th century when Yoga was introduced to the Western hemisphere from its Indian homeland, it has undergone various adaptations. Today, Yoga is practiced in five major ways:

- ✔ As a method for physical fitness and health maintenance
- ✔ As a sport
- ✔ As body-oriented therapy
- ✔ As a comprehensive lifestyle
- ✔ As a spiritual discipline

We take a look at these five basic approaches in the upcoming sections.

Yoga as fitness training

The first approach, Yoga as fitness training, is the most popular way that Westerners practice Yoga. It's also the most radical revamping of traditional Yoga. More precisely, it's a revision of traditional *Hatha Yoga.* Yoga as fitness training is concerned primarily with the physical body — its flexibility, resilience, and strength. This is how most newcomers to Yoga encounter this great tradition.

Fitness training is certainly a useful gateway into Yoga, but later on, some people discover that Hatha Yoga also includes moral and spiritual practices that are designed to lead to enlightenment. From the earliest times, Yoga masters have emphasized the need for a healthy body. But they've also always pointed beyond the body to the mind and other important aspects of being.

Yoga as a sport

This second approach, Yoga as a sport, is especially prominent in some Latin American countries but is widely controversial. Its practitioners, many of whom are excellent athletes, master hundreds of extremely difficult Yoga postures to perfection and demonstrate their skills and beautiful physiques in international competitions.

But this new sport, which also can be regarded as an art form, has drawn much criticism from the ranks of more traditional Yoga practitioners. They feel that competition has no place in Yoga. Yet this athletic orientation has done much to put Yoga on the map in some parts of the world.

We see nothing wrong with good-natured Yoga competitions as long as self-centered competitiveness is held in check.

Yoga as therapy

The third approach, Yoga as therapy, applies yogic techniques to restore health or full physical and mental functioning. In recent years, some Western Yoga teachers have begun to use yogic practices for therapeutic purposes.

Although the idea behind Yoga therapy is very old, its name is fairly new. Yoga therapy is, in fact, a whole new professional discipline, calling for far greater training and skill on the part of the teacher than is the case with ordinary Yoga.

Commonly, Yoga is intended for those who don't suffer from disabilities or ailments requiring remedial action and special attention. Yoga therapy, on the other hand, addresses these special needs. For example, Yoga therapy may be able to help you find relief from certain ailments such as chronic back pain, asthma, rheumatism, and many others.

 Seeing the potency of Yoga therapy, several insurance companies now offer coverage for it as a part of their alternative therapies programs. Other insurance companies will no doubt follow suit before long. If you're looking for a certified Yoga therapist, contact the International Association of Yoga Therapists at 928-541-0004 or go to www.iayt.org.

Yoga as a lifestyle

The fourth approach, Yoga as a lifestyle, enters the proper domain of Yoga. Yoga once or twice a week for an hour or so is certainly better than no Yoga at all. And Yoga can be enormously beneficial even when practiced only as fitness training.

But you unlock the real potency of Yoga when you adopt it as a lifestyle. This means *living* Yoga; practicing Yoga every day, whether it's physical exercises or meditation. Above all, it means applying the wisdom of Yoga to everyday life and to live lucidly (that is, with awareness). Yoga has much to say about what and how you should eat, how you should sleep, how you should work, how you should relate to others, and so on. It offers a total system of conscious and skillful living.

Don't think that you have to be a yogic superstar to practice lifestyle Yoga. You can begin today. Just make a few simple adjustments in your daily schedule and keep your goals vividly in front of you. Whenever you're ready, make further positive changes — one step at a time.

Yoga as a spiritual discipline

Lifestyle Yoga is concerned with healthy, wholesome, functional, and benevolent living. Yoga as a spiritual discipline, the fifth and final approach, is concerned with all that *plus* the traditional ideal of *enlightenment* — that is, discovering your spiritual nature.

The word *spiritual* has been abused a lot lately, so we need to explain how it's used here. *Spiritual* relates to *spirit* — your ultimate nature. In Yoga, it is called the *atman* (pronounced *aht-mahn*) or *purusha (poo-roo-shah)*.

According to Yoga philosophy, the *spirit* is one and the same for everyone. It's formless, immortal, superconscious, and unimaginably blissful. It is one and the same in all beings and things. It is transcendental because it exists beyond the limited body and mind. You discover the spirit in the moment of your enlightenment.

What all approaches to Yoga have in common

The five approaches to Yoga share at least two *fundamental practices:* the cultivation of awareness and relaxation.

✔ **Awareness** is the peculiarly human ability to pay close attention to something, to be consciously present, to be mindful. Yoga is attention training.

To see what we mean, try this exercise: Pay attention to your right hand for the next 60 seconds. That is, feel your right hand and do nothing else. Chances are, your mind is drifting off after only a few seconds. Yoga consists in reining in your attention whenever it strays.

> ✔ **Relaxation** is the conscious release of unnecessary and, therefore, unwholesome tension in the body.

Both awareness and relaxation go hand in hand in Yoga. Without bringing awareness and relaxation to Yoga, the exercises would be merely exercises — not *yogic* exercises.

Conscious breathing is often added to awareness and relaxation as a third foundational practice. Normally, breathing happens automatically. In Yoga, awareness is brought to this act, which then makes it into a powerful tool for training the body and the mind. We say much more about these aspects of Yoga in Chapter 4.

Empowering Yourself with Yoga

Outside agents like physicians, therapists, or remedies can help us through major crises, but we ourselves are primarily responsible for our own health and happiness. Especially the source of lasting happiness lies within us. Yoga reminds us of this truth and helps us mobilize the inner strength to live responsibly and wisely.

Maintaining health and happiness

What is health? Most people answer this question by saying that health is the opposite of illness. But health is *more* than the absence of disease. It's a positive state of being. Health is wholeness. To be healthy means not only to possess a well-functioning body and a sane mind but also to vibrate with life, to be vitally connected with one's social and physical environment. To be healthy also means to be happy.

Finding out what being healthy really means

 Because life is constant movement, you shouldn't expect health to be static. Perfect health is a mirage.

In the course of your life, you can expect inevitable fluctuations in your state of health — even cutting your finger with a knife temporarily upsets the balance. Your body reacts to the cut by mobilizing all the necessary biochemical forces to heal itself.

Regular Yoga practice can create optimal conditions for self-healing. You achieve a baseline of health, with an improved immune system that enables you to stay healthy longer and heal faster.

Healing rather than curing

Yoga is about healing rather than curing. Like a really good physician, Yoga takes deeper causes into account. These causes, more often than not, are to be found in the mind, in the way you live. That's why Yoga masters recommend self-understanding.

Taking an active role in your own health

Most people tend to be passive in health matters. They wait until something goes wrong, and then they rely on a pill or a physician to fix the problem. Yoga encourages you to take the initiative in preventing illness and restoring or maintaining your health.

Something for nothing?

The computer industry has coined thousands of new terms. One is particularly relevant to Yoga practice: *gigo,* which means "garbage in, garbage out." It captures a simple truth: The quality of a cause determines the quality of the effect. In other words:

✔ Don't expect health from junk food.

✔ Don't expect happiness from miserable attitudes.

✔ Don't expect good results from shoddy Yoga practice.

✔ Don't expect something from nothing.

Yoga is a powerful tool, but you must learn to use it properly. You can buy the latest super-duper computer, but if you only know how to use it as a typewriter, that's all it is. You get out of Yoga what you put into it.

Keep an open mind. Allow yourself to be surprised by Yoga's comprehensiveness. Don't settle for *just* this or that. Even after decades of Yoga practice and study, we're still discovering new things about Yoga.

Taking control of your health has nothing to do with self-doctoring (which can be dangerous); it's simply a matter of taking responsibility for your health. A good physician will tell you that healing is greatly facilitated when the patient actively participates in the process. For example, you may take various kinds of medication to deal with a gastric ulcer, but unless you learn to eat well, sleep adequately, avoid stress, and take life more easy, you're bound to have a recurrence before long. You must change your lifestyle.

Following your bliss

Yoga suggests that the best possible meaning you can find for yourself springs from the well of joy deep within you. That joy or bliss is the very nature of the spirit, or transcendental Self (refer to "Yoga as a spiritual discipline," earlier in this chapter). Joy is like a 3-D lens that captures life's bright colors and motivates you to embrace life in all its countless forms. Yoga points the way to happiness, health, and life-embracing meaning.

Realizing Your Human Potential with Yoga

Don't put a ceiling on your own potential and growth! In 1865, Richard Webster ran 1 mile in 4:36.5. In 1993, Noureddine Morceli took only 3:44.39 to do the same. At the first Olympic Games in Athens in 1896, Ellery Clark reached 5 feet 11.25 inches in the running high jump event. A century later, at the Olympic Games in Atlanta, Georgia, Charles Austin improved the record to 7 feet 10 inches. The story is similar for other sports.

You may never be a world-class athlete. You (and we) are, however, *in principle* capable of anything that great Yoga masters can do. We all share the same human potential. Whether you actualize it depends largely on how determined you are and whether you find the right method for tapping into your own inner strength and wisdom.

Yoga makes good use of the mind, which is an incredible resource. Don't ask us to define what the mind is. We'd have to answer in the words of a comedian and say, "It doesn't matter." (When asked what matter is, the same comedian replied, "Never mind.") When speaking about the mind, we usually mean the mental attitudes that shape your behavior.

Although Yoga is mind training, it isn't *just* mind training. It includes the physical body, which Yoga views as a great treasure. Having a body provides you with valuable experiences and lessons, and the body is the foundation on which you build your entire life. Yoga asks you to take proper care of your body through reasonable diet and physical exercise, as well as appropriate rest and sleep. At the same time, Yoga tells you that you're not *just* the body but also the mind, and not *just* the mind but also a greater "something" beyond body and mind — what we call the *spirit.*

Balancing Your Life with Yoga

Hindu tradition explains Yoga as the discipline of balance. This is another way of expressing the ideal of unity through Yoga. Everything in you must harmonize to function optimally. A disharmonious mind is disturbing in itself, but sooner or later, it also causes physical problems. An imbalanced body can easily warp your emotions and thought processes. If your relationships with others are strained, you cause distress not only for them but for yourself as well. And when your relationship to your physical environment is disharmonious, well, you trigger serious repercussions for everyone.

A beautiful and simple Yoga exercise called "The Tree" is meant to improve your sense of balance and promote your inner stillness. Even when conditions force a tree to grow askew, it always balances itself out by growing a branch in the opposite direction in which it's forced to lean. In this posture, you stand still like a tree, perfectly balanced.

Yoga helps you apply this principle of balance to your life. Whenever life's demands and challenges force you to bend to one side, your inner strength and peace of mind serve as counterweights. Rising above all adversity, you can never be uprooted.

 The tree posture improves overall balance, stability, and poise. It strengthens the legs, arms, and shoulders, and "opens" (relaxes and loosens up) the hips and groin. The posture, like the other one-leg balancing poses, enhances focus and concentration and produces a calming effect on the body and mind.

1. **Stand in the mountain posture (see Chapter 5).**

2. **As you exhale, bend your left knee and place the sole of your left foot, toes pointing down, on the inside of your right leg between your knee and your groin.**

3. **As you inhale, bring your arms over your head and join your palms together.**

4. **Soften the arms and focus on a spot 6 to 8 feet in front of you on the floor (see Figure 1-1).**

   Stay in Step 4 for 6 to 8 breaths and then repeat with the opposite leg.

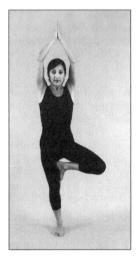

Figure 1-1: The tree posture improves your sense of balance.

Chapter 2

Prep Before Pep

• •

In This Chapter

▶ Approaching Yoga with a healthy attitude

▶ Leaving the competition behind

▶ Translating your own mind-body language

▶ Doing it your way without regret

• •

*I*n Yoga, *what* you do and *how* you do it are equally important — and both mind and body contribute to your actions. Yoga respects the fact that you are not merely a physical body but a psychophysical *body-mind.* Full mental participation in even the simplest of physical exercise enables you to tap into your deeper potential as a human being.

This chapter is about the right attitude toward practice, especially the yogic postures, which is the best preparation for success in Yoga. Among other things, we examine the spirit of competitiveness, which has no place in Yoga. We encourage you to find your own pace, without pushing yourself and risking injury. We also express the importance of function over form, proposing that you modify the "ideal" form of an exercise to suit your specific needs.

Remember: Yoga is not a military drill but a creative endeavor that asks you to call on the formidable powers of your own mind as you explore and enjoy yogic possibilities.

Cultivating the Right Attitude

Your attitudes reveal a lot about you and your social background. Attitudes are enduring tendencies in your mind, which show themselves not only in your speech but also in your behavior. Yoga encourages you to examine all your basic attitudes about life to discover which ones are wrong and dysfunctional so that you can replace them with better, more appropriate attitudes.

One of the attitudes worth cultivating is balance in everything. A balanced attitude in this context means that you're willing to build up your Yoga practice step by step instead of expecting instant perfection. It also means not basing your practice on wrong assumptions, including the mistaken notion that Yoga is about tying yourself in knots. On the contrary, Yoga tries to loosen all our physical, emotional, and intellectual knots.

Pretzels are not us!

Many people are turned off when they see publications featuring photographs of adept practitioners in advanced postures, with their limbs tied into knots.

Those publications sometimes neglect to tell you that most of the people in the photographs have practiced Yoga several hours a day for many years to achieve their level of skill. Trust us! You don't have to be a pretzel to experience the undeniable benefits of Yoga.

In Yoga sports — one of five orientations we mention
in Chapter 1 — more than 2,000 postures are possible.
Many of these postures call for such great strength and
flexibility that only a top gymnast could perform them
flawlessly. The postures certainly look beautiful and
intriguing when mastered, but their health benefits are
the same as the 20 or so fundamental postures that
make up most practitioners' daily routines.

So, unless you aim to participate in Yoga competitions,
you won't have to worry about all those glamorous-
looking postures you may find in some books and mag-
azines or on colorful posters. Most of these postures
are new inventions, whereas Yoga masters have been
content for centuries with just a handful of practices
that have stood the test of time.

Practice at your own pace

People who are natural pretzels are typically double-
jointed. If you're not inherently noodle-like, you can
expect to have to practice regularly to increase your
body's flexibility and muscular strength.

We advocate a graduated approach. The late Yoga
master T. Krishnamacharya of Madras, India, who is
the source of most of the best-known orientations of
modern Hatha Yoga, expressed the importance of tai-
loring Yoga instruction to the needs of each individual. He recommended that Yoga teachers take a
student's age, physical ability, emotional state, and
occupation into account — we agree completely. So,
our best advice to you is basic and simple: Proceed
gently, but steadfastly.

 If you like to learn Yoga from books, choose
them carefully. Especially look closely at
whether the exercise descriptions include all
the stages of developing comfort with a particular posture. To ask a middle-aged newcomer to

Yoga to imitate the final form of many of the postures without providing suitable transitions and adaptations is a prescription for disaster. Don't worry — this book emphasizes exercises that are both feasible and safe.

Send the scorekeeper home

Americans often grow up in a highly competitive environment. From childhood on, we're encouraged to do more, push harder, and secure success. In sports like football, basketball, and soccer, young players are indoctrinated with the spirit of competitiveness. Although competition has its place in society, elbowing your way to victory can be harmful to yourself and others. And this type of competitive behavior has no place in the practice of Yoga.

Many years ago, a middle-aged man came to one of our classes. He was a friendly enough fellow but extremely competitive and hard on himself. Right away, he announced that he was intent on mastering the lotus posture within a few weeks and pushed himself during our classes. We cautioned him repeatedly to proceed more slowly. After only a few visits, he failed to show up and never returned. Later, we learned from a mutual friend that he had asked his wife to sit on his legs to force them into the lotus posture. Her weight had seriously injured both of his knees!

Yoga is about peace, tranquility, and harmony — the exact opposite of the competitive mindset. Yoga doesn't require you to fight against anyone, least of all yourself, or to achieve some goal by force. On the contrary, you're invited to be kind to yourself and others and, above all, to collaborate with rather than coerce your body or do battle with your mind. Yoga is gentle. In its gentleness, however, it is extremely powerful.

No pain, no gain — Not!

 The idea of "no pain, no gain" — a completely mistaken notion — often reinforces competitiveness. Yoga doesn't ask you to be a masochist. Pain and discomfort are part of life, but this realization doesn't require you to invite them. On the contrary, the goal of Yoga is to overcome all suffering. Therefore, never flog your body; always only coax it gently. Our motto is: No gain from pain.

Enjoying a Safe and Sound Yoga Practice

As you travel through yogic postures, you begin to build awareness of the communications taking place between your body and mind. Do you feel peacefully removed from the raging storm of life around you, comfortable and confident with your strength, motion, and steadiness? Or are you painfully in tune with the passage of time, sensing a physical awkwardness or strain in your movements?

Listening to your own rhythms — and acknowledging their importance — can help make your Yoga experience an expression of peace, calm, and security. And that positive message is what Yoga practice is all about.

Debunking the myth about "perfect" posture

 Some modern schools of Hatha Yoga claim that they teach "perfect" postures that you can slip into as easily as a tailor-made suit. But how can a perfect posture exist when we're all different? Should a 15-year-old athlete perform a posture

or an entire postural routine following the same
guidelines that apply to a 60-year-old retiree?
Surely not. Besides, these schools disagree
among themselves about what constitutes a perfect posture. So, to spell it out, the perfect posture is perfectly mythical.

Posture, as explained by the great Yoga master
Patanjali 2,000 years ago, has only two requirements:
A posture should be *steady* and *comfortable.* What
could be more plain and simple? Although Patanjali
was thinking primarily — perhaps even exclusively —
in terms of meditation postures, his formula applies
to all postures equally.

✔ **Steady posture:** A steady posture is a posture
that's held stable for a certain period of time. The
key isn't freezing all movement, though. Your posture becomes steady when your mind is steady.
As long as your thoughts run wild and your negative emotions are not held in check, your body
also remains unsteady. As you become more
skilled in self-observation, you begin to notice the
ever-revolving carousel of your mind and become
sensitive to the tension in your body. That tension
is what Yoga means by "unsteadiness."

✔ **Comfortable posture:** A posture is comfortable
when it is enjoyable and enlivening rather than
boring and burdensome. A comfortable posture
increases the principle of clarity — *sattva* — in
you. But please don't confuse comfort with
slouching. *Sattva* and joy are intimately connected. The more *sattva* is present in your body-
mind, the more relaxed and happy you'll be.

Listening to your body

No one knows your body like you do. The more you
practice Yoga, the better you can become at deter-
mining your limitations with each posture: Each

posture presents its own unique challenge. Ideally, you want to feel encouraged to explore and expand your physical and emotional boundaries without risking strain or injury to yourself.

Some teachers speak of practicing at the edge. The *edge* is the point of intensity where a posture challenges you but doesn't cause you pain or unusual discomfort. The idea is to gradually — very slowly and carefully — push that edge farther back and open up new territory. To be able to practice at the edge, you must cultivate self-observation and pay attention to the feedback from your body.

Each Yoga session is an exercise in self-observation without being judgmental. Listen to what your body is telling you through its ongoing communications. Signals constantly travel from your muscles, tendons, ligaments, bones, and skin to your brain. Train yourself to become aware of them. You want to be in dialogue with your body instead of indulging in a monologue that focuses on your own mind without awareness of your body. Pay particular attention to signals coming from the neck, lower back, jaw muscles, abdomen, and any known problem areas of your body.

To gauge the intensity of a difficult Yoga posture, use a scale from 1 to 10, with 10 being at the threshold of pain. Imagine a flashing red light and an alarm bell going off after you pass level 8. Notice the signals and heed them. Especially watch your breath. If your breathing becomes labored, it's usually a good indication that, figuratively speaking, you're going over the edge. ***Remember:*** You are the world's foremost expert on what your body is trying to tell you.

Beginners commonly experience trembling when holding certain Yoga postures. Normally, the involuntary motion is noticeable in the legs or arms and is nothing to worry about, as long as you aren't straining. The tremors are simply a sign that your muscles are working in response to a new demand. Instead of focusing on the feeling that you've become a wobbly bowl of jelly, make your breath a little longer if you can and allow your attention to go deeper within. If the trembling starts to go off the Richter scale, you need to either ease up a little or end the posture altogether.

Moving slowly but surely

All postural movements are intended for slow performance. Unfortunately, most of the time, we're on automatic. Our movements tend to be unconscious, too fast, and not particularly graceful. We stumble, bump into things, and are generally unaware of our bodies. The yogic postures oblige you to adopt a different attitude.

Here are some of the advantages of slow motion:

- ✔ **You enhance your awareness,** which enables you to *listen* to what your body is telling you and to practice at the *edge* (see the preceding section).

- ✔ **You lower the risk of straining or spraining muscles, tearing ligaments, or overtaxing your heart.** In other words, your practice becomes much safer.

- ✔ **You experience relaxation more quickly.**

- ✔ **You don't get out of breath, and your breathing overall is improved.**

- ✔ **You enable more muscle groups to come into action to share the workload.**

For the best results, practice your postures at a slow, steady pace while calmly focusing on your breath and the postural movement (see Chapter 4). Resist the temptation to speed up; instead, savor each posture. Remember to relax and be present here and now. If your breathing becomes a little bit labored or you begin to feel fatigued, just rest until you're ready to go on.

 If you find yourself rushing through your program, pause and ask yourself why you're in a hurry. If you have an actual reason, such as an imminent appointment, your best bet is to crop your program by focusing on fewer exercises. If you can't shake the feeling of being pressured by time, you may want to postpone your Yoga session altogether and practice conscious breathing (see Chapter 4) while you go about your other business.

 However, if you're rushing through your program because you're feeling bored or distracted for some other reason, pause and remind yourself why you're practicing Yoga in the first place. Renew your motivation by telling yourself that you have plenty of time to complete your session; you have no earthly reason to be in any hurry. Boredom is a sign that you're detached from your own bodily experience and you're not living in the present moment. Resume your Yoga practice as a full participant in the process. If you need more than a mental reminder, use one of the relaxation techniques that we describe in Chapter 3 to slow yourself down. As we explain in Chapter 4, full yogic breathing in one of the resting postures also has a wonderful calming effect.

Practicing function over form with Forgiving Limbs

In Yoga, as in life, function is more important than form. Beginners, in particular, need to adapt postures to enjoy the function and benefits of a given posture early in their practice experiences.

We call one very useful adaptive device *Forgiving Limbs.* With Forgiving Limbs, you give yourself permission to slightly bend your legs and arms instead of keeping them fully extended. You don't need to feel like a wimp if you're kind to your body in order to help yourself achieve the function of a posture. Although bent arms and legs don't look flashy, they enable you to move your spine more easily, which is the focus of many postures and the key to a healthy spine.

 For example, the primary mechanical function of a standing forward bend is to stretch your lower back. If you have a good back, take a moment to see what we mean in this adapted posture that's safe for beginners:

1. **Stand up straight and, *without forcing anything,* bend forward and try to place your head on your knees with the palms of your hands on the floor (see Figure 2-1a).**

   Very few men or women can actually do this, especially beginners.

2. **Now stand up again, separate your feet to hip width, and bend forward, allowing your legs to bend until you can place your hands on the floor and almost touch your head to your knees (see Figure 2-1b).**

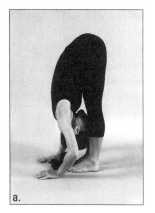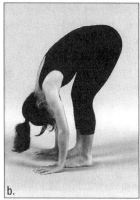

Figure 2-1: Classic form (a) and modified form with Forgiving Limbs (b).

As you become more flexible — and you will! — gradually straighten your legs until you can come closer to the ideal posture. A common lower back injury occurs when weekend warriors, inspired by young, nubile instructors, try to do the seated version of the straight-legged forward bend and push too far.

Remember: Bending your legs and arms to achieve the intended function of a posture is perfectly all right. Especially for beginners, bending is safer than attempting to achieve the final form.

Approaching exercise with open eyes

 Many Yoga conferences entertain the question of whether you should keep your eyes open or closed during Yoga practice. In a nutshell, if you're comfortable with your eyes closed, then we recommend that you close them. You may feel more focused and able to hear your body's signals. However, standing and balancing postures require you to keep your eyes open.

With a little practice, you can stay focused even with your eyes open. In general, Yoga favors an open-eyed approach to life's challenges. The yogis and yoginis like to know what's in front of them, so many seasoned practitioners also execute the postures with open eyes.

Seasoned meditators, by the way, can enter into deep meditation without shutting their eyes, though don't be surprised if they have a blank look; they have effectively withdrawn their awareness from external reality and are happily conscious at a different level. You can expect to experience something of this attitude as you master the various postures and breathing exercises.

Chapter 3

Relaxed like a Noodle: The Fine Art of Letting Go of Stress

. . . .

In This Chapter

▶ Understanding the nature of stress

▶ Relaxing the body

▶ Acquiring a calm mind

. . . .

*L*ife in general — not merely modern life — is inherently stressful. Even an inanimate object, such as a rock, experiences an element of stress. Not all stress is bad for you, however. The question is whether that stress is helping you or killing you.

Psychologists distinguish between *distress* and *eustress* (good stress). Yoga can help you minimize distress and maximize good, life-enhancing stress. For example, a creative challenge that stimulates your imagination and fires your enthusiasm, but that doesn't cause you anxiety or lost sleep, is a positive event. Even a joyous celebration is, strictly speaking, stressful; but the celebration's not the kind of stress that kills you — at least not in modest doses. On the other hand, doing nothing and feeling bored to tears is a form of negative stress.

In this chapter, we talk about how you can control negative stress not only through various yogic-relaxation techniques, but also by cultivating appropriate attitudes and habits.

The Nature of Stress

Stress is a fact of life. Some estimates indicate that 80 percent of all illnesses result from stress. Endocrinologist Hans Selye, who pioneered research on stress, distinguished three phases of the stress syndrome: alarm, resistance, and exhaustion. *Alarm* can be a harmless activity like stepping from a warm house into the cold air or receiving an upsetting phone call. Both situations require the body to make an adjustment, which is a kind of *resistance.* When the demand on the body goes on for too long, the stage of *exhaustion* sets in, which can lead to a complete breakdown of the body and the mind — be it heart disease, high blood pressure, failure of the immune system, or mental illness.

Bad stress creates an imbalance in the body and the mind, causing you to tense your muscles and breathe in a rapid and shallow manner. Under stress, your adrenal glands work over-time and your blood becomes depleted of oxygen, which starves your cells. Constant stress triggers the fight-or-flight response, putting you in a chronic state of alertness that's extremely demanding on your body's energies.

Because of the relentless demands that modern life makes on us — work, noise, pollution, and so on — most people experience chronic stress. How can you deal with it efficiently? Yoga suggests a three-pronged solution:

✔ Correct those attitudes that are stress-producing.

✔ Change habits that invite stress into your life.

✔ Release existing tension in the body and do so on an ongoing basis.

Stress can occur without any unpleasant stimulus. Even a birthday celebration can cause you stress, usually because of some hidden anxiety (like another year to mark off). Stress is cumulative and can creep up on you so gradually that it's imperceptible — until its acute and adverse symptoms manifest.

Correcting wrong attitudes

Yoga's integrated approach works with both the body and the mind, offering potent antidotes to just the sort of attitudes that make you prone to stress, especially egotism, extreme competitiveness, perfectionism, and the sense of having to accomplish everything right now and by yourself. In all matters, Yoga seeks to replace negative thoughts and attitudes with positive mental dispositions. Yogic practice helps you understand that everything has its proper place and time. Yoga asks you to be kind to yourself.

If you, like so many stress sufferers, have a hard time asking for help, Yoga can give you a real appreciation that we are all interdependent. If you are, by nature, distrustful of others, Yoga puts you in touch with that part of your psyche that naturally trusts life itself. It shows you that you don't need to feel as if you were under attack, because your real life — your spiritual identity — can never be harmed or destroyed.

Wherever ego, I go

The ultimate source of stress is the ego, or what the Yoga masters call the "I-maker" *(ahamkara),* from *aham* ("I") and *kara* ("maker"). From the perspective of Yoga, the ego is a mistaken notion in which we identify with our particular body rather than the universe as a whole. Consequently, we experience fear of death and attachment to the body and the mind. This attachment, which is the survival instinct, in turn gives rise to all those many emotions and intentions that make up the game of life. Keeping this artificial center — the ego — going is inherently stressful. The Yoga masters all agree that by relaxing the grip of the ego, you can experience greater peace and happiness.

Changing poor habits

Everything in the universe follows an ebb-and-flow pattern that you can count on. Seasons change, and newborn babies eventually become elderly adults. Yogic wisdom recommends that you adopt the same natural patterns into your personal life. You may spend much of your time being serious, but you need to play, too. In fact, you need to make time to *just be* with no expectations and no guilt. Taking time to *just be* is good for your physical and mental health. Work and rest, tension and relaxation belong together as balanced pairs.

Often, people desperately maintain a hectic schedule because they can't envision an alternative that includes time out. They fear what may happen if they were to slow down. But money and standard of living aren't everything, and the *quality* of your life is far more important. Besides, if stress undercuts your health, you have to go into low gear anyway, and your climb back to health may prove very costly. Yoga gives you a baseline of tranquility to deal with your fears effectively.

Your inner wisdom tells you that your body and mind are subject to change and that nothing in your environment permanently stays the same. Therefore, there's no point in anxiously clinging to anything. Yoga recommends that you constantly remember your spiritual nature, which is beyond the realm of change and ever blissful. However, Yoga also asks you to care for others and the world you live in, but all the while appreciating that you can't step into the same river twice.

 Of course, you can do many practical things, which are described in books on stress management, to reduce stressful situations. These suggestions include not waiting until the last minute to start or finish projects, improving your communication with others, avoiding confrontations, and accepting that we live in an imperfect world.

 Your daily Hatha Yoga routine, especially the relaxation exercises, can help you extend the feeling of peacefulness or calmness beyond the session to the rest of the day. Pick some activities or situations that you repeat several times a day — such as when you go to the bathroom, wait at a traffic light, sit down, open or close a door, look at your watch, or hang up the telephone — and use these as reminders to consciously relax. Whenever you encounter these activities, exhale deeply and consciously relax, remembering the peaceful feeling evoked in your daily session.

Detach yourself

Yoga shows you how to cultivate the *relaxation response* throughout the day by letting go of your hold on things. This phrase was coined by Herbert Benson, MD, who was among the first to point out the hidden epidemic of *hypertension* (high blood pressure) as a result of stress. In his national bestseller *The Relaxation Response,* he calls the relaxation response "a universal human capacity" and "a remarkable innate, neglected asset."

Yoga teaches you how to tap into that underused capacity of your own body-mind. The yogic equivalent of the relaxation response is *vairagya,* which means literally "dispassion" or "nonattachment." It's good to feel passionate about what you do rather than have a lukewarm attitude. At the same time, however, you merely invite suffering when you become too attached to people, situations, and the outcome of your actions. Yoga recommends an attitude of inner detachment in all matters. This detachment doesn't spring from boredom, failure, fear, or any neurotic attitude but from inner wisdom.

For example, if you're a mother, you'll love and take tender care of your children. But if you also are a *yogini,* you won't succumb to the stress-producing illusion that you *own* your children. Instead, you always remain aware of the fact that your sons and daughters have their own lives to live, which may turn out to be quite different from yours, and that all you can do is guide them as best you can.

Releasing bodily tension

 Yoga pursues tension release through all its many different techniques, including breathing exercises and postures, but especially relaxation techniques. The former are a form of *active* or *dynamic relaxation;* the latter are a form of *passive* or *receptive relaxation.*

Relaxation Techniques That Work

The Sanskrit word for relaxation is *shaithilya,*
which is pronounced *shy-theel-yah* and means
"loosening." It refers to the loosening of bodily
and mental tension — all the knots that you tie
when you don't go with the flow of life. These
knots are like kinks in a hose, which prevent the
water from flowing freely.

Keeping muscles in a constant alert state expends a
great amount of your energy, which then is unavail-
able when your muscles are called upon to really
function. Conscious relaxation trains your muscles to
release their grip when you don't use them. This
relaxation keeps the muscles responsive to the signals from your brain telling them to contract so that
you can perform all the countless tasks of a busy day.

Tips for a successful relaxation practice

Relaxation is not quite the same as doing nothing.
Often, when we believe we're doing nothing, we're
really busy contracting unused muscles — quite
unconsciously. Relaxation is a conscious endeavor that
lies somewhere between effort and noneffort. To truly
relax, you have to understand and practice the skill.

Relaxation doesn't require any gadgets, but you
may try the following:

✔ Practice in a quiet environment where you're
  unlikely to be disturbed by others or the
  telephone.

✔ Try placing a small pillow under your head and
  a large one under your knees for support and
  comfort in the *supine,* or lying, positions.

✔ Ensure that your body stays warm. If necessary, heat the room first or cover yourself with a blanket. Particularly avoid lying on a cold floor, which isn't good for your kidneys.

✔ Don't practice relaxation techniques on a full stomach.

Deep relaxation: The corpse posture

The simplest and yet the most difficult of all Yoga postures is the corpse posture (*shavasana,* from *shava* and *asana,* pronounced *shahvah ah-sah-nah*), also widely known as the dead pose (*mritasana,* from *mrita* and *asana*). This posture is the simplest because you don't have to use any part of your body at all, and it's the most difficult precisely because you're asked to do nothing whatsoever with your limbs. The corpse posture is an exercise in mind over matter. The only props you need are your body and mind.

Here's how you do the corpse pose (see Figure 3-1):

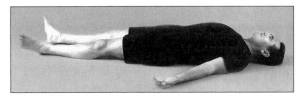

Figure 3-1: The corpse is the most popular of all Yoga poses.

1. **Lie flat on your back, with your arms stretched out and relaxed by your sides, palms up (or whatever feels most comfortable).**

Place a small pillow under your head if you need one and another large pillow under your knees for added comfort.

2. **Close your eyes.**

3. **Form a clear intention to relax.**

   Some people find it helpful to picture themselves lying in white sand on a sunny beach.

4. **Take a couple of deep breaths, lengthening exhalation.**

5. **Contract the muscles in your feet for a couple of seconds, and then consciously relax them.**

   Do the same with the muscles in your calves, upper legs, buttocks, abdomen, chest, back, hands, forearms, upper arms, shoulders, neck, and face.

6. **Periodically scan all your muscles from your feet to your face to check that they are relaxed.**

   You can often detect subtle tension around the eyes and the scalp muscles. Also, relax your mouth and tongue.

7. **Focus on the growing bodily sensation of no tension, and let your breath be free.**

8. **At the end of the session, before opening your eyes, form the intention to keep the relaxed feeling for as long as possible.**

9. **Open your eyes, stretch lazily, and get up slowly.**

Practice 10 to 30 minutes; the longer the duration, the better.

Allowing relaxation to end on its own is best — your body knows when it has benefited sufficiently and naturally brings you out of relaxation. However, if you have only a limited time for the exercise, set your mental clock to

that time after closing your eyes as part of your
intention. If you need to have a sound to remind
you to return to ordinary waking consciousness,
make sure that your wristwatch or clock isn't so
loud that it startles you and provokes a heavy
surge of adrenaline.

Afternoon delight

When your energies flag in the afternoon, try the
following exercise, which is a great stress
buster. You can practice it at home or in a quiet
place at the office — just make sure that you
won't be interrupted. For this exercise, you
need a chair, one or two blankets, and a towel
or an eye bag. Allow five to ten minutes.

1. **Lie on your back and put your feet up on the
   chair, which should face you (see Figure 3-2).**

   Make sure that your legs and back are comfortable. Your legs should be 15 to 18 inches apart.
   You can also put your legs and feet up on the edge
   of a bed. If none of the feet-up positions feels good,
   just lie on your back with your legs bent and feet
   placed on the floor. If the back of your head is not
   flat on the floor, and your neck and throat feel
   tense, or if your chin is pushed up toward the ceiling, raise your head slightly on a folded blanket or
   firm, flat cushion to feel comfortable.

2. **Cover your body from the neck down with one
   of the blankets.**

   Don't let your body cool down too quickly, which
   can not only feel uncomfortable and interfere
   with your relaxation, but also cramp your muscles and harm your kidneys.

3. **Place the eye bag or towel folded lengthwise
   over your eyes.**

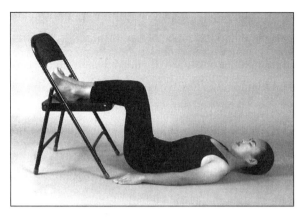

Figure 3-2: Inhale freely, and then exhale forever.

4. **Rest for a few moments, and get used to the position.**

5. **Visualize a large balloon in your stomach. As you inhale through your nose, expand the imaginary balloon in all directions. As you exhale through your nose, release the air from the balloon.**

   Repeat several times until the exercise becomes easy for you.

6. **Now inhale freely and begin to make your exhalation longer and longer.**

   Inhale freely, exhale forever.

7. **Repeat at least 30 times.**

8. **When you finish the exercise, allow your breath to return to normal and rest for a minute or so, enjoying the relaxed feeling.**

   Don't rush getting up.

Magic triangles

The following relaxation technique again utilizes your power of imagination. If you can picture things easily in your mind, you'll find the exercise enjoyable and refreshing. For this exercise, you need a chair and a blanket (if necessary). Allow five minutes.

1. **Sit up tall in a chair, with your feet on the floor and comfortably apart and your hands resting palms up on top of your knees (see Figure 3-3).**

   If your feet are not comfortably touching the floor, fold up the blanket and place it under your feet for support.

2. **Breathe through your nose, but allow your breath to move freely.**

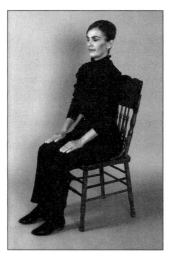

Figure 3-3: Mentally focus on the part of the triangle that is hard to connect.

3. **Close your eyes and focus your attention on the middle of your forehead, just above the level of your eyebrows.**

   Make sure that you don't crinkle your forehead or squint your eyes.

4. **Visualize as vividly as possible a triangle connecting the forehead point and the palms of both hands.**

   Register (but don't think about) any sensations or colors that appear on your mental screen while you're holding the triangle in your mind. Do this for 8 to 10 breaths and then dissolve the triangle.

5. **Visualize a triangle formed by your navel and the big toes of your feet.**

   Retain this image for 10 to 12 breaths. If any part of the mental triangle is difficult to connect, persist in focusing on that part until the triangle fully forms.

6. **This final step is more challenging: Keeping your eyes closed, visualize again the first triangle formed between your forehead and your two palms.**

   When you have a clear image, visualize at the same time the second triangle formed between your navel and your big toes. Picture both triangles together for 12 to 15 breaths, and then dissolve them.

Relaxation before sleep

If you want to enjoy deep sleep or you're experiencing insomnia (but don't want to count sheep), the following exercise can help you. Many people don't make it to the end of this relaxation technique without falling asleep. For this exercise, you need the following props: a bed or other comfortable place to sleep, two pillows, and one or two blankets. Allow five to ten minutes.

1. **Prepare yourself for sleep and get into bed, lying on your back under the blankets.**

   Your legs can be straight or bent at the knees with your feet flat on the mattress.

2. **Place one pillow under your head and have the other one close by.**

3. **With your eyes closed, begin to breathe through the nose, making your exhalation twice as long as your inhalation.**

   Keep your breathing smooth and effortless. Also, don't try to direct your breath to any part of your body. Let the 1:2 breathing ratio be effortless, something you can keep up.

4. **Remain on your back for eight breaths; then roll over onto your right side and place the second pillow between your knees. Now use the same 1:2 ratio for 16 breaths.**

5. **Finally, roll over onto your left side, with the second pillow still between your knees, and use the 1:2 ratio for 32 breaths.**

Yogic Sleep (Yoga Nidra)

Yogic Sleep is a very powerful relaxation technique that you can do after you gain some control over the relaxation response. When practiced successfully, this technique is as restorative as sleep — except you remain fully aware throughout.

Its traditional name — *yoga nidra* (pronounced *yoh-gah nee-drah*) — makes reference to Brahma, the Hindu creator god, who "sleeps"

between successive world creations. His sleep is never unconscious.

One feature of this practice is to focus in relatively quick succession on individual parts of the body (as described later). Mentally name each part and then feel it as distinctly as possible.

In the beginning, you may find it difficult to actually feel certain body parts. Don't let this dismay you, but continue to rotate your awareness fairly rapidly. Later, as you become more skilled at this technique, you can slow down the rotation and feel each part ever more distinctly. With practice, you can include in this circuit even the inner organs.

Practicing Yoga Nidra before sleep is best because it's an excellent technique for inducing lucid dreaming and out-of-the-body experiences during sleep. *Lucid dreaming* refers to the kind of dream in which you're aware that you're dreaming. Great Yoga masters remain aware even during deep sleep. Only the body and brain are fast asleep, whereas awareness is continuous.

Here is how you perform Yoga Nidra:

1. **Lie flat on your back, with your arms stretched out by your sides, palms up, or whatever feels most comfortable (refer to Figure 3-1).**

   Place a pillow behind your neck for support and another pillow under your knees for added comfort.

2. **Close your eyes.**

3. **Form a clear intention.**

4. **Take a couple of deep breaths, emphasizing exhalation.**

5. **Starting with your right side, rotate your awareness through all parts of the body — limb by limb — in fairly quick succession: each finger, palm of the hand, back of the hand, the hand as a whole, forearm, elbow, upper arm, shoulder joint, shoulder, neck, each section of the face (forehead, eyes, nose, chin, and so on), ear, scalp, throat, chest, side of the rib cage, shoulder blade, waist, stomach, lower abdomen, genitals, buttocks, whole spine, thigh, top and back of knee, shin, calf, ankle, top of foot, heel, sole, each toe.**

6. **Be aware of your body as a whole.**

7. **Repeat the rotation one or more times until adequate depth of relaxation is achieved, always ending with whole-body awareness.**

8. **Be aware of the whole body and the space surrounding it.**

   Feel the stillness and peace.

9. **Reaffirm your initial intention.**

10. **Mentally prepare to return to ordinary consciousness.**

11. **Gently move your fingers for a few moments, take a deep breath, and then open your eyes.**

No time limit applies to your Yoga Nidra performance, unless you impose one. Expect to come out of Yogic Sleep naturally, whether you return after only 15 minutes or a whole hour. Or you may just fall asleep. So if you have things to do afterward, make sure you set your wristwatch or clock for a *gentle* wakeup call.

Yoga Nidra over mind

Using the Yoga Nidra technique serves as a potent tool for reprogramming your brain because you can reach a deep level of the mind. This deep-level reaching is done by formulating an intention. The Sanskrit word for intention is *samkalpa* (pronounced *sahm-kahl-pah*), meaning *intention, desire, wish,* or *will*. An intention may be your aspiration to become enlightened for the benefit of all beings; your wish to overcome anger, jealousy, unkindness, or any other negative emotion; or simply your desire to become or remain healthy. Be sincere about your intention and repeat it at least a dozen times both at the beginning and the end of the exercise.

Chapter 4

Breath and Movement Simplified

*T*he masters of Yoga discovered the usefulness of the breath thousands of years ago and in Hatha Yoga have perfected a system for the conscious control of breathing. In this chapter, we share their secrets with you. In the ancient Sanskrit language, the word for *breath* is the same as the word for *life* — *prana* (pronounced *prah-nah*) — which gives you a good clue about how important Yoga thinks breathing is for your well-being.

Breathe Your Way to Good Health

Think of your breath as your most intimate friend. Your breath is with you from the moment you're born and stays with you until you die. In a given day, you take between 20,000 and 30,000 breaths. Most likely, though — barring any respiratory problems — you're barely aware of your breathing. This is like taking your best friend for granted in such a way that the relationship gets stale and is put at risk. To be sure, allowing breathing to occur automatically isn't necessarily to your advantage, because automatic doesn't always mean optimal. In fact, most people's breathing habits are quite poor and to their great disadvantage. They accumulate a lot of stale air in their lungs, which become as unproductive as a stale friendship. Poor breathing is known to cause and increase stress. Conversely, stress shortens your breath and increases your level of anxiety.

You can help alleviate stress through the simple practice of yogic breathing. Among other things, breathing loads your blood with oxygen, which, by nourishing and repairing your body's cells, maintains your health at the most desirable level. Shallow breathing, which is widespread, doesn't oxygenate the 10 pints of blood circulating in your arteries and veins very efficiently. Consequently, toxins pile up in the cells. Before you know it, you feel mentally sluggish and emotionally down, and eventually organs begin to malfunction. Is it any wonder that the breath is the best tool you have to profoundly affect your body and mind?

In Yoga, consciously regulated breathing has the following three major applications:

- ✔ Use it in conjunction with the various postures to achieve the deepest possible effect and to prepare the mind for meditation.

- ✔ Use it as breath control (called *pranayama,* pronounced *prah-nah-yah-mah*), to invigorate your vitality.

✔ Use it as a healing method, in which you consciously direct the breath to a particular part or organ of the body to remove energetic blockages and facilitate healing; this is Yoga's gentle version of acupuncture.

Taking high-quality breaths

Before you jump right in and make drastic changes to your method of breathing, take a few minutes to assess your current breathing style. You may find it helpful to keep a log of your breathing habits over the course of a couple of days, noting how your breathing changes as situations around you occur.

Check your breathing by asking yourself the following questions:

✔ Is my breathing shallow (my abdomen and chest barely move when I fill my lungs with air)?

✔ Do I often breathe erratically (my breathing rhythm is not harmonious)?

✔ Do I easily get out of breath?

✔ Is my breathing labored at times?

✔ Do I generally breathe too fast?

If your answer to any of these questions is yes, you make an ideal candidate for yogic breathing. Even if you didn't answer yes, practicing conscious breathing still benefits your mind and body.

By the way, men take an average of 12 to 14 breaths per minute, while women take 14 to 15. Breathing at a markedly faster pace — usually associated with *chest breathing* — qualifies as hyperventilation, which leads to carbon dioxide depletion. (Your body needs some of this gas to maintain the right acid-alkaline balance of the blood.)

Relaxing with a couple of deep breaths

Think about the many times you've heard someone say "Now just take a couple of deep breaths and relax." This recommendation is so popular because it really works! Pain clinics across the country use breathing exercises for pain control. Childbirth clinics teach Yoga-related breathing techniques to both parents to aid the birthing process. Moreover, since the 1970s, "stress gurus" have taught yogic breathing to corporate America with great success.

 One easy way to experience the effect of simple breathing is to try the following exercise:

1. **Sit comfortably in your chair.**

2. **Close your eyes and visualize a swan gliding peacefully across a crystal-clear lake.**

3. **Now, like the swan, let your breath flow along in a long, smooth, and peaceful movement. Ideally, inhale and exhale through your nose.**

   If your nose is plugged up, try the combination of nose and mouth, or just the mouth.

4. **Extend your breath to its comfortable maximum for 20 rounds; then gradually let your breath return to normal.**

5. **Afterward, take a few moments to sit with your eyes closed and notice the difference in how you feel overall.**

Can you imagine how relaxed and calm you would feel after 10 to 15 minutes of conscious yogic breathing?

Practicing safe yogic breathing

 As you look forward to the calming and restorative power of yogic breathing, take time to reflect on a few safety tips that can help you enjoy your experience.

- ✔ If you have problems with your lungs (such as a cold or asthma), or if you have a heart disease, consult your physician first before embarking on breath control even under the supervision of a Yoga therapist.

- ✔ Don't practice breathing exercises when the air is too cold or too hot.

- ✔ Avoid practicing in polluted air, including the smoke from incense; whenever possible, practice breath control outdoors or with an open window.

- ✔ Don't strain your breathing — remain relaxed while doing the breathing exercises.

- ✔ Don't overdo the number of repetitions. Stay within our guidelines for each exercise.

- ✔ Don't wear any constricting pants or belts.

Reaping the benefits of yogic breathing

In addition to relaxing the body and calming the mind, yogic breathing has an entire spectrum of other benefits that work like insurance, protecting your investment in a longer and healthier life. Here are six important gains of controlled breathing:

- ✔ It steps up your metabolism (the best manager of weight increase).

- ✔ It uses muscles that automatically help improve your posture so that you can prevent the stiff, slumped carriage characteristic of many older people.

✔ It keeps the lung tissue elastic, which allows you to take in more oxygen food for the 50 trillion cells in your body.

✔ It tones your abdominal area, which is a common site for health problems, because many illnesses begin in the intestines.

✔ It helps strengthen your immune system.

✔ It reduces your levels of tension and anxiety.

Breathing through the nose

No matter what anybody else tells you, yogic breathing is typically done through the nose, both during inhalation and exhalation. For the traditional yogis and yoginis, the mouth is meant for eating and the nose for breathing. We know at least three good reasons for breathing through the nose:

✔ It slows down the breath because you're breathing through two small openings instead of the one big opening in your mouth. Slow is good in Yoga.

✔ The air is hygienically filtered and warmed by the nasal passages. Even the purest air contains at least dust particles and at worst all the toxic pollutants of a metropolis.

✔ According to traditional Yoga, nasal breathing stimulates the subtle energy center — the so-called *ajna-cakra* (pronounced *ah-gyah-chuk-rah*), which is located near sinuses in the spot between the eyebrows. This very important location is the meeting place of the left (cooling) and the right (heating) current of vital energy *(prana)* that act directly on the nervous and endocrine systems.

Folk wisdom knows that every rule has an exception, which is definitely the case with the yogic rule of breathing through the nose. A few classical yogic techniques for breath control require you to breathe through the mouth. When presenting a mouth-breathing technique, we alert you to that fact.

 You may suffer from various physiological conditions that prevent you from breathing through the nose. Of course, Yoga is flexible. If you have difficulty breathing when lying down, try sitting up. The time of day can also make a difference in your ability to breathe. For example, you may be more congested or allergic in the morning than in the afternoon. You can detect the differences. If you're still not sure how to settle on a comfortable breathing method, first try inhaling through the nose and exhaling through the mouth and, failing this, just breathe through your mouth and don't worry for now. Worry is always counterproductive.

 In the beginning, save yogic breathing for your Yoga exercises. Down the line, when you become more skillful at it, you may want to adopt nasal breathing during all normal activities. You can then benefit from its calming and hygienic effects throughout the day.

The Mechanics of Yogic Breathing

Most people are either shallow-chest breathers or shallow-belly breathers. Yogic breathing incorporates a complete breath that expands both the abdomen and the chest on inhalation either from the abdomen up or the chest down. Both are valid techniques.

Yogic breathing involves breathing much deeper than usual, which in turn brings more oxygen into your system. Don't be surprised if you feel a little lightheaded or even dizzy in the beginning. If this happens during your Yoga practice, just rest for a few minutes or lie down until you feel like proceeding. Remind yourself that there's no rush.

 Some Yoga practitioners think that it is the breath that flows either down into the chest or upward. Not so. The breath obviously always comes from above (either the nose or the mouth) and then expands into the lungs, depending on the contraction of the muscles in the upper torso. Any suggestion of an up or down movement of the breath is due entirely to the sequence of your muscular control and the flow of your attention.

In both chest and abdominal breathing, the abdomen draws in on exhalation. From a mechanical standpoint, Yoga breathing moves the spine and works the muscles and organs of respiration, which primarily include the diaphragm, *intercostal* (between the ribs) and abdominal muscles, and the lungs and heart. When the diaphragm contracts, it is pulled down, which creates more space for the lungs during inhalation. The chest noticeably widens. When the diaphragm relaxes, it moves back into its upward curve, forcing the air out of the lungs.

 The *diaphragm* is a vaulted muscle sheath that separates the lungs and heart from the stomach, liver, kidneys, and other abdominal organs. It is attached all around the lower border of the rib cage and, by a pair of powerful muscles, to the first through fourth lumbar vertebrae. The diaphragm and the chest muscles activate the lungs, which don't have muscles themselves.

The diaphragm and your emotions

Psychologically, people tend to use the diaphragm as a "lid" by which they bottle up their "undigested" or unwanted emotions of anger and fear. Chronic contraction of the diaphragm makes it inflexible and blocks the free flow of energy between the abdomen and the chest (the nether region of the bowels and the feelings associated with the heart). Yogic breathing helps restore flexibility and function to the diaphragm and removes obstructions to the flow of psychosomatic energy (the life force). You can then experience liberation of your emotions, which can lead you to integrate them with the rest of your life.

Deep breathing not only affects the organs in your chest and abdomen, but also reaches down into your "gut" emotions. Don't be surprised if sighs and perhaps even a few tears accompany the tension release your breath work achieves. These are welcome signs that you are peeling off the muscular armor you have placed around your abdomen and heart. Instead of feeling concerned or embarrassed, rejoice in your newly gained inner freedom!

Appreciating the complete yogic breath

If shallow or erratic breathing put your well-being at risk, the complete yogic breath is your ticket to excellent physical and mental health. If you do no other Yoga exercise, the complete Yoga breath— integrally combined with relaxation — will still be of inestimable benefit to you. It's your secret weapon, except Yoga doesn't believe in the use of force.

Before you jump into practicing the complete yogic breath, try out this belly breathing exercise:

1. **Lie flat on your back and place one hand on your chest, the other on your abdomen (see Figure 4-1).**

   Place a small pillow or folded blanket under your head if you have tension in your neck or if your chin tilts upward. Place a large pillow under your knees if your back is uncomfortable.

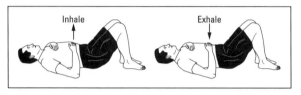

Figure 4-1: Belly breathing exercises the diaphragm and prepares you for the complete yogic breath.

2. **Take 15 to 20 slow, deep breaths.**

   During inhalation, expand your abdomen; during exhalation, contract your abdomen — but keep your chest as motionless as possible. Your hands will act as motion detectors.

3. **Pause for a couple of seconds between inhalation and exhalation, keeping the throat soft.**

In belly-to-chest breathing, shown in Figure 4-2, you really exercise your chest and diaphragm muscles, as well as your lungs, and treat your body with oodles of oxygen and *prana* (life force). Your cells will be humming with energy and your brain will be very grateful to you for the extra boost. You can use this form of breathing before you begin your relaxation practice, before and where indicated during your practice of the Yoga postures, and whenever you feel so inclined throughout the day. You don't necessarily have to lie down, as stipulated for the following exercise. You can be seated or even walking. After practicing this technique for a while, you may find that it's become second nature to you.

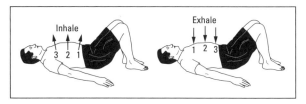

Figure 4-2: This is the classic Yoga breath.

1. **Lie flat on your back with your knees bent and feet on the floor at hip width. Relax.**

   Place a small pillow or folded blanket under your head if you have tension in your neck or if your chin tilts upward. Place a large pillow under your knees if your back is uncomfortable.

2. **Inhale while expanding the abdomen, and then the ribs, and finally the chest.**

   Pause for a couple of seconds.

3. **Exhale while releasing chest and shoulder muscles, gently and continuously contracting or drawing the abdomen in.**

   Pause again for a couple seconds.

4. **Repeat the sequence.**

You can greatly enhance the value of this and other exercises by fully participating with your mind. *Feel* the air fill your lungs. *Feel* your muscles work. *Feel* your body as a whole. *Visualize* precious life energy entering your lungs and every cell of your body, rejuvenating and energizing you. To help you experience this exercise more profoundly, keep your eyes closed. You also can place your hands on your abdomen and feel it expand upon inhalation.

Classically, yogic breathing was taught from the abdomen up on inhalation, which you can see in numerous publications on Yoga. This method works very well for a lot of people. However, in the 1960s, Yoga master T. K. V. Desikachar, with the guidance of his father, the late T. Krishnamacharya, began to adapt the traditional yogic breathing to the needs of their Western students.

Think about it! In the West, we sit in chairs and bend forward too much. Our daily sitting routine begins in the early morning when we go to the bathroom. Then we lean over the sink to brush our teeth and do whatever else we do to our faces. We sit at the breakfast table, and then we sit again while we commute to our workplace. At work we clock a lot more time sitting, perhaps slouching, in front of a computer or bending over a machine. Finally, in the evening, we come home and sit down for dinner and afterward, perhaps, sit in front of the television or our computer until our eyes get blurry.

The chest-to-belly breathing emphasizes arching the spine and the upper back to compensate for all this bending forward throughout the day, and it also works very well for moving in and out of Yoga postures. Chest-to-belly breathing is also an excellent energizer in the morning and can be done even before you hop out of bed. We don't recommend this exercise late at night, though, because it's likely to keep you awake.

 The chest-to-belly breathing exercise (shown in Figure 4-3) complements the belly-to-chest breathing (refer to Figure 4-2). As with the belly-to-chest breathing technique, you can practice the following exercise lying down or while you're walking.

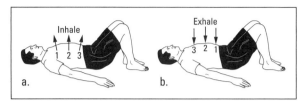

Figure 4-3: The new Yoga breath.

1. **Lie flat on your back, with your knees bent and feet on the floor at hip width. Relax.**

   Place a small pillow or folded blanket under your head if you have tension in your neck or if your chin tilts upward. Place a large pillow under your knees if your back is uncomfortable.

2. **Inhale while expanding the chest from the top down and continuing this movement downward into the belly (see Figure 4-3a).**

   Pause for a couple of seconds.

3. **Exhale while gently contracting and drawing the belly inward, starting just below the navel (see Figure 4-3b).**

   Pause for a couple of seconds.

4. **Repeat the sequence.**

Starting out with focus breathing for beginners

If you're having a little difficulty synchronizing yourself with the rhythm of the complete Yoga breathing techniques, you may want to start with a simpler method we call *focus breathing*. Focus breathing is a great stepping stone to all

the other techniques and may be just what you
need for a confidence-builder.

During your Yoga practice, simply follow the directions we give you about when to inhale and exhale for
each posture, breathe only through the nose and
make the breath a little longer than normal. That's all
you have to do! Don't worry about where the breath
is starting or ending, just breathe slowly and evenly.

After you're used to this practice, just add a short
pause of 1 or 2 seconds after inhalation and another
pause after exhalation.

When you're comfortable with these practices, add
drawing the belly in during exhalation — without
force or exaggeration.

Taking a pause

During your normal shallow breathing, you'll notice a
slight natural pause between inhalation and exhalation.
This pause becomes very important in yogic breathing.
Even though the duration is usually only 1 or 2 seconds,
this pause is a natural moment of stillness and meditation. If you pay attention to this pause, it can help you
become more aware of the unity between body, breath,
and mind — all of which are key elements in your Yoga
practice. With the help of a teacher, you also can learn
to lengthen the pause during various Yoga postures to
heighten its positive effects.

Partners in Yoga: Breath
and Postural Movement

In Hatha Yoga, breathing is just as important as the
postures. How you breathe when you're moving into,

holding, or moving out of any given posture can greatly increase the efficiency and the benefits of your practice.

Here are some basic guidelines:

- ✔ **Let the breath surround the movement.** The breath leads the movement by a couple of seconds; that is, you initiate breathing (both inhalation and exhalation), and then you make the movement. When you inhale, the body opens or expands; when you exhale, the body folds or contracts.

- ✔ **Both inhale and exhale end with a natural pause.**

- ✔ **In the beginning, let the breath dictate the length of the postural movement.** For example, if you're raising your arms as you inhale and you run out of breath before you reach your goal, just pause your breathing for a moment and then bring your arms back down as you exhale. With practice, your breath will gradually get longer.

- ✔ **Let the breath itself be your teacher.** When your breath sounds labored, it's time to back off or come out of a posture.

- ✔ **Try to sense the breath flowing into the area you're working with any given posture.**

Breathing in four directions

You can move your body in four natural directions:

- ✔ **Flexion:** Bending forward.
- ✔ **Extension:** Bending backward.

✔ **Lateral flexion:** Bending sideways.

✔ **Rotation:** Twisting your body.

Normally, when people move they tend to hold or strain their breath. In Yoga, you simply follow the natural flow of the breath. As a rule, adopt this pattern:

✔ Inhale when moving into back bends (as shown in Figure 4-4a).

✔ Exhale when moving into forward bends (see Figure 4-4b).

✔ Exhale when moving into side bends (see Figure 4-4c).

✔ Exhale when moving into twists (as shown in Figure 4-4d).

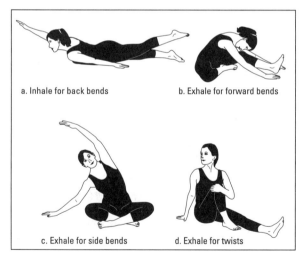

a. Inhale for back bends

b. Exhale for forward bends

c. Exhale for side bends

d. Exhale for twists

Figure 4-4: Breathing properly during postures is important.

Combining breath with movement

Most Yoga books talk about *stationary* or *held* Yoga postures *(asanas)*. We suggest that before learning to hold a posture, you first become acquainted with moving in and out of most of the postures we recommend in this book. Always, of course, follow the rules of breath and movement given in the preceding section on inhalation and exhalation. Then, when you can move in and out of a given posture easily and confidently, try holding the posture for a short period *without* retaining or straining your breath. You can tell you're straining when your face is turning into a grimace or you feel it going red like a tomato.

We note the number of repetitions and how long to hold them in all our recommended programs. With practice, you develop an idea of what's right for you.

We often ask you to hold a posture for 6 to 8 breaths, which translates to roughly 30 seconds. Keep breathing when you hold a posture — don't hold your breath.

Now and then, we still see eager Yoga practitioners seeking to achieve better flexibility by bouncing during the holding phase of a stretching posture. This practice is part of old-school training, which is really not such a good habit after all. Bouncing not only tends to disconnect you from the breath but also can be risky, especially if your muscles are stiff or not adequately warmed up. Be kind to yourself!

The arrows in the following exercise and wherever they appear in this book tell you the direction of postural movement and the part of the breath that goes with the movement. *Inhale*

means inhalation; *exhale* means exhalation;
breaths means the number of breaths defining
the length of a postural hold.

1. **Lie on your back comfortably, with your legs
   straight or bent.**

   Place your arms at your sides near your hips with
   the palms turned down (see Figure 4-5a).

2. **Inhale through your nose. After 1 or 2 seconds,
   begin to slowly raise your arms up over your
   head — in sync with inhalation — until they
   touch the ground behind you (see Figure 4-5b).**

   Leave your arms slightly bent.

3. **When you reach the end of inhalation, pause
   for 1 or 2 seconds even if your arms don't make
   it to the floor. Then exhale slowly through your
   nose and bring your arms back to your sides
   along the same path (as in Step 1).**

4. **Repeat this movement with a nice slow rhythm.**

   Remember: Open or expand as you inhale; fold
   or contract as you exhale.

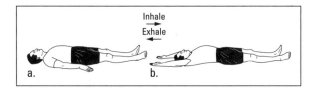

Figure 4-5: The breath surrounds the movement.

After you become comfortable with this exercise, combine it with each of our recommended breathing techniques: Use either focus breathing (refer to "Starting

out with focus breathing for beginners" earlier in this chapter), belly breathing (refer to Figure 4-1), belly-to-chest breathing (refer to Figure 4-2), or chest-to-belly breathing (refer to Figure 4-3). You can decide which technique you prefer as you begin combining breathing with movement.

Chapter 5

Recommended Routines

● ●

In This Chapter

▶ Keeping current on basic Yoga principles

▶ Presenting an eight-week beginners' plan

● ●

*I*f you follow the plan in this chapter diligently, you can improve your flexibility, muscle tone and strength, and concentration. Very likely, you'll notice a number of other benefits as well, such as better stamina, digestion, and sleep. As the adage says, all beginnings are difficult. True enough, but we make your first steps in Hatha Yoga as simple as possible. Now you just need to take the first step — and then the next.

✔ **Weeks 1 and 2:** Use Beginner 1, Part I (about 15 minutes per session) a minimum of three times per week to a maximum of six times per week.

✔ **Weeks 3 and 4:** Use Beginner 1, parts I and II (about 30 minutes) a minimum of three times per week to a maximum of six times per week.

✔ **Weeks 5 and 6:** Use Beginner 2, Part I, and Beginner 1, Part II (approximately 30 minutes) a minimum of three times per week to a maximum of six times per week.

✔ **Weeks 7 and 8:** Use Beginner 2, parts I and II (about 30 minutes) a minimum of three times per week to a maximum of six times per week.

When practicing the various postures that we describe in the following sections, either follow the directions for breath and movement or simply stay in each posture for six to eight breaths.

Because this may be your first Yoga experience — and you may have turned directly to this chapter — we offer a quick trip through some basic principles:

✔ **Yoga is not competitive.** Be patient. If you follow the directions, you will improve over time no matter what your starting level.

✔ **Move slowly into and out of the postures.** Don't ever rush your Yoga session. Coming out of a posture is an integral part of the posture itself.

✔ **Use yogic breathing throughout the routine (see Chapter 4).**

✔ **Pause briefly after each inhalation and exhalation (see Chapter 4).**

✔ **Challenge but don't strain yourself.** Yoga should never hurt or cause you pain.

✔ **Move smoothly into and out of a posture several times before holding the posture.** Doing so prepares your body for a deeper stretch and helps you concentrate on linking the body, breath, and mind.

✔ **Don't change the order of the sequence and just randomly pick the postures that you want.** All the routines have a special order or sequence to give you the maximum benefits.

Beginner 1, Part 1

You can use this routine as a 15-minute, stand-alone routine, or you can combine it with the Beginner 1,

Part II routine for a 30-minute session. We include the necessary warm-up and compensation postures, as well as rest.

If you have time only for a 15-minute session, we recommend that you practice the exercises in this section rather than the ones in Part II.

Corpse posture

1. **Lie flat on your back with your arms relaxed along the sides of your torso, palms up (see Figure 5-1).**

2. **Inhale and exhale through your nose slowly for eight to ten breaths.**

   Pause briefly after each inhalation and exhalation. Use focus breathing (see Chapter 4) in this posture and for the rest of this routine.

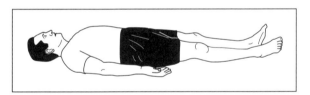

Figure 5-1: First relax, and then use focus breathing for the rest of this routine.

Lying arm raise

1. **Lie in the corpse posture, arms relaxed at your sides, palms down (see Figure 5-2a).**

2. **As you inhale, slowly raise your arms up overhead and touch the floor behind you (see Figure 5-2b).**

   Pause briefly.

3. **As you exhale, bring your arms back to your sides as in Step 3.**

4. **Repeat Steps 2 and 3 six to eight times.**

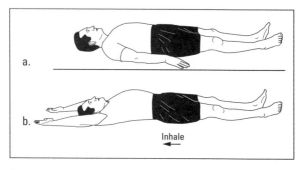

Figure 5-2: Link the breath and movement from the very beginning.

Knee-to-chest posture

1. **Lie on your back, knees bent, feet flat on the floor.**

2. **As you exhale, bring your right knee into your chest and extend your left leg down.**

   Hold your shin just below your knee (see Figure 5-3). If you have knee problems, hold the back of your thigh instead.

3. **Stay in Step 2 for six to eight breaths, and then repeat on the left side.**

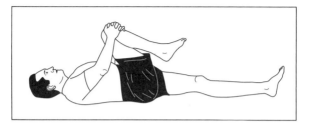

Figure 5-3: Prepare the lower body and tune each side of the back.

Downward-facing dog

1. **Beginning on your hands and knees, place your hands directly under your shoulders, palms spread on the floor, with your knees directly under the your hips**

   Straighten your arms, but don't lock your elbows (see Figure 5-4a).

2. **As you exhale, lift and straighten (but don't lock) your knees.**

   As your hips lift, bring your head down to a neutral position so that your ears are between your arms (see Figure 5-4b). If possible, press your heels to the floor and your head toward your feet (stop if doing so strains your neck).

3. **As you inhale, come back down to your hands and knees as in Step 1.**

4. **Repeat Steps 1 through 3 three times; and then stay in Step 2 for six to eight breaths.**

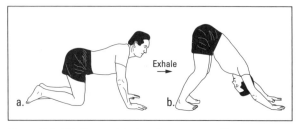

Figure 5-4: This first weight-bearing posture will prepare you for the main standing postures.

Child's posture

1. **Starting on your hands and knees, place your knees about hip width apart, hands just below your shoulders.**

   Your elbows are straight but not locked.

2. **As you exhale, sit back on your heels; rest your torso on your thighs and your forehead on the floor. (You don't have to sit all the way back.)**

3. **Lay your arms back on the floor beside your torso, palms up, or reach your relaxed arms forward, palms on the floor.**

4. **Close your eyes and stay in the folded position for six to eight breaths (see Figure 5-5).**

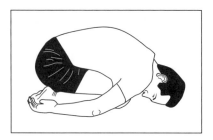

Figure 5-5: A short rest before the most physical part of the routine.

Warrior posture

1. **Stand in the mountain posture (see Figure 5-15, later in this chapter). As you exhale, step forward about 3 to 3½ feet (or the length of one leg) with your right foot.**

   Turn your left foot out (so the toes point to the left) if you need more stability.

2. **Place your hands on the top of your hips and square the front of your pelvis.**

   Then release your hands and hang your arms (see Figure 5-6a).

3. **As you inhale, raise your arms forward, overhead and bend your right knee to a right angle, so that your knee is directly over your ankle and your thigh is parallel to the floor (see Figure 5-6b).**

4. **Soften your arms (see Chapter 2 for a description of Forgiving Limbs) and face your palms toward each other.**

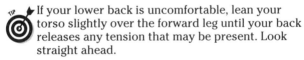

If your lower back is uncomfortable, lean your torso slightly over the forward leg until your back releases any tension that may be present. Look straight ahead.

5. **Repeat Steps 3 and 4 three times, and then hold once on the right side for six to eight breaths.**

6. **Repeat the same sequence on the other (left) side.**

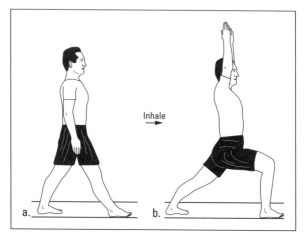

Figure 5-6: Imagine that you're a warrior — a symbol of power and strength.

Standing forward bend

1. **Start in the mountain posture (refer to Figure 5-15, later in this chapter). As you inhale, raise your arms forward, and then up overhead (see Figure 5-7a).**

2. **As you exhale, bend forward from the hips.**

   When you feel a pull in the back of your legs, soften your knees (see Chapter 2 for information about Forgiving Limbs) and hang your arms (see Figure 5-7b).

   If your head is not close to your knees, bend your knees more. If you have the flexibility, straighten your knees while keeping them soft. Relax your head and neck downward.

3. **Exhaling, roll the body up like a rag doll stacking the vertebra one at a time.**

4. **Repeat Steps 1 through 3 three times; and then stay down in Step 2 for six to eight breaths.**

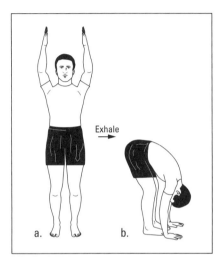

Figure 5-7: You're not a wimp if you soften your knees.

Reverse triangle posture

1. **Stand in the mountain posture (see Figure 5-15, later in this chapter). As you exhale, step out to the right about 3 to 3½ feet (or the length of one leg) with the right foot.**

2. **As you inhale, raise your arms out to the sides, parallel to the line of your shoulders and the floor, so that your shoulders form a T with your torso (see Figure 5-8a).**

3. **As you exhale, bend forward from the hips and then place your right hand on the floor near the inside of your left foot.**

4. **Raise your left arm toward the ceiling and look up at your left hand.**

   Soften your knees and arms. Bend your left knee or move your right hand away from your left foot and more directly under your torso, if you experience strain or discomfort (see Figure 5-8b).

5. **Repeat Steps 2 through 4 to the same side three times; then stay down in Step 4 for six to eight breaths.**

6. **Repeat the same sequence on the right side.**

You can strengthen or strain your neck in this posture. Turn your neck down if you're uncomfortable.

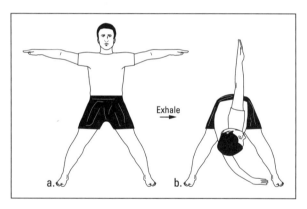

Figure 5-8: This standing twist will rejuvenate your entire spine.

Standing spread leg forward bend

1. **Stand in the mountain posture (see Figure 5-15 later in this chapter). As you exhale, step out to the right about 3 to 3½ feet (or the length of one leg) with your right foot.**

2. As you inhale, raise your arms out to the sides parallel to the line of your shoulders and the floor, so that your shoulders form a T with the torso (see Figure 5-9a).

3. As you exhale, bend forward from the hips and soften your knees.

4. Hold your bent elbows with the opposite-side hands and hang your torso and arms.

5. Stay folded in this posture for six to eight breaths (see Figure 5-9b).

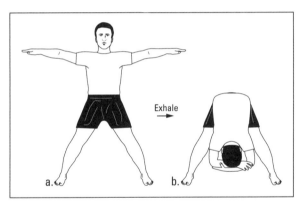

Figure 5-9: Just hang comfortably. Notice each time how close you get to the floor.

The karate kid

1. Stand in the mountain posture (see Figure 5-15, later in this chapter). As you inhale, raise your arms out to the sides parallel to the line of your shoulders and the floor, so that your shoulders form a T with the torso.

2. **Steady yourself and focus on a spot on the floor 10 to 12 feet in front of you.**

3. **As you exhale, bend and raise your left knee toward the chest, keeping your right leg straight (see Figure 5-10).**

4. **Stay in Step 3 for six to eight breaths.**

5. **Repeat with your legs reversed.**

After you become stable in the karate kid posture, extend your left leg down toward the floor, keeping your foot slightly off the floor. Then gradually, over time, raise your left leg higher and higher until it's parallel with the floor. Try this added step on both sides.

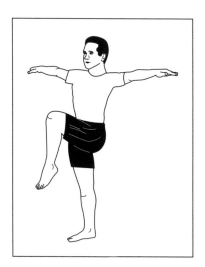

Figure 5-10: Remember this posture from a famous movie?

Corpse posture

Repeat the corpse posture exercise, as described at the beginning of this routine (refer to Figure 5-1). Stay for six to eight breaths.

If you're in the first two weeks of your practice, stop here. If you've been practicing longer than two weeks, you're now at the halfway point, or approximately 15 minutes, of your routine. You may stop here or continue for the next 15 minutes to complete a 30-minute session.

Beginner 1, Part II

This routine expands on the exercise sequence of "Beginner 1, Part I." The sequences have the same level of difficulty. If you only have time for a 15-minute session rather than a full 30 minutes, we recommend that you use the exercises of Beginner 1, Part I rather than the following exercises.

Yogi sit-up

1. Lie on your back, knees bent, feet on the floor at hip width.

2. Turn your toes in "pigeon-toed" and touch your inner knees together.

3. Spread your palms on the back of your head, fingers interlocked, and hook your thumbs under the angle of the jawbone, just below the ears (see Figure 5-11a).

4. As you exhale, press your knees firmly (but without causing yourself discomfort), tilt the front of your pelvis toward your navel, and, with your hips on the floor, slowly sit up halfway.

Keep your elbows out to the sides in line with the tops of your shoulders. Look toward the ceiling (see Figure 5-11b). Don't pull your head up with your arms; instead, support your head with your hands and come up by contracting the abdominal muscles.

5. **As you inhale, slowly roll back down.**

6. **Repeat Steps 4 through 6 six to eight times.**

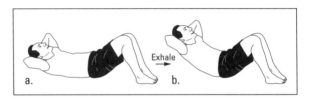

Figure 5-11: Exhale as you sit up. Keep your eyes on the ceiling.

Cobra 2

1. **Lie flat on your belly, separate your legs to hip width and point your toes back with the tops of your feet on the floor.**

2. **Bend your elbows and place your palms on the floor with your thumbs near your armpits.**

   Put your forehead on the floor and relax your shoulders (see Figure 5-12a).

3. **As you inhale, begin to raise your chest and head. When you feel the muscles of your lower back engaging, press your hands down and arch your spine until you're looking straight ahead (see Figure 5-12b).**

   Keep the top-front hip bones on the floor and your shoulders dropped away from your ears. Unless you're very flexible, keep your elbows slightly bent.

4. **As you exhale, lower your torso and head slowly back to the floor.**

5. **Repeat Steps 3 and 4 three times; then hold in the up position for six to eight breaths.**

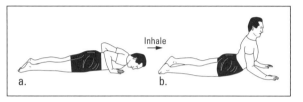

Inhale

a.   b.

Figure 5-12: Lift your chest only as high as you feel comfortable.

Child's posture

Refer to Figure 5-5. Close your eyes and stay in the folded position for six to eight breaths.

Hamstring stretch

1. **Lie on your back, legs straight. Place your arms along your sides, palms down.**

2. **Bend just your left knee and put your left foot on the floor (see Figure 5-13a).**

3. **As you exhale, bring your right leg up as straight as possible (see Figure 5-13b).**

4. **As you inhale, return your leg to the floor, keeping your head and the back of your pelvis on the floor.**

5. **Repeat Steps 3 and 4 three times; then hold your right leg with your hands interlocked on the back of your raised thigh, just above your knee, for six to eight breaths (see Figure 5-13c).**

6. **Repeat on the left side.**

 Lift your head on a pillow or folded blanket if
the back of your neck or your throat tenses
while raising or lowering the leg.

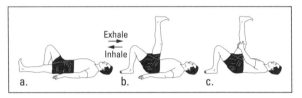

Figure 5-13: Stretching your hamstrings will help you to
improve many postures.

Head-to-knee posture

1. **Sitting on the floor with your legs stretched out
   in front of you, bend your left knee and bring
   your left foot toward your right groin.**

2. **Bring your bent left knee down to the floor on
   the left side (but don't force it), and place the
   sole of your left foot on the inside of the right
   thigh, heel in the groin.**

   The toes of your left foot point toward the right
   knee.

3. **Bring your back up nice and tall and, as you
   inhale, raise your arms forward and up overhead until they're beside your ears.**

   Keep your arms and the right leg soft and slightly
   bent in Forgiving Limbs, as we describe in
   Chapter 2 (see Figure 5-14a).

4. **As you exhale, bend forward from your hips,
   bringing your hands, chest, and head toward
   your right leg.**

   Rest your hands on your leg, knee, or foot. If your
   head is not close to your right knee, bend your
   knee more until you feel your back stretching on
   the right side (see Figure 5-14b).

5. **Repeat Steps 3 and 4 three times. Then stay
   folded in Step 4 for six to eight breaths.**

6. **Repeat the same sequence on the opposite side.**

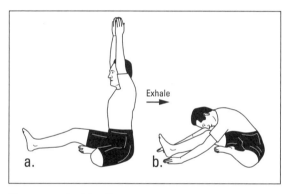

Exhale

a.   b.

Figure 5-14: Avoid pulling yourself down. Just relax in the posture and breathe.

Corpse posture

To perform this posture, refer to Figure 5-1 in
the "Corpse posture" section. Stay for eight to
ten breaths.

Beginner 2, Part 1

After four weeks of practicing the exercises that we describe in Parts I and II of the Beginner 1 series, you're probably ready to move on to the slightly more challenging postures of Beginner 2. If you don't feel quite ready yet, however, continue to practice the Beginner 1 exercises for a few more weeks or for as long as necessary to achieve competence in the postures. Take your time — no one is rushing you.

This routine is either a 15-minute stand-alone routine, or you can combine it with the Beginner 1, Part II routine for a 30-minute session (in weeks 5 and 6 of our eight-week program) or the Beginner 2, Part II routine for a 30-minute session (in weeks 7 and 8 of our eight-week program).

Mountain posture

1. **Stand tall but relaxed with your feet at hip width.**

2. **Hang your arms at your sides, palms turned toward your legs.**

3. **Visualize a vertical line connecting the hole in your ear, your shoulder joint, and the sides of your hip, knee, and ankle.**

4. **Look straight ahead, eyes open or closed (see Figure 5-15).**

5. **Use the three-part yogic breathing or chest-to-belly breathing (see Chapter 5) for eight to ten breaths, and then continue with that breathing pattern for the entire routine.**

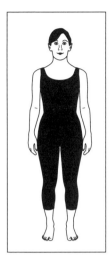

Figure 5-15: Starting with this first pose, keep a union with your body, breath, and mind.

Rejuvenation sequence

1. **Stand in the mountain posture with your feet at hip width and arms at your sides (see Figure 5-16a).**

2. **As you inhale, slowly raise your arms out from the sides and up overhead (see Figure 5-16b). Pause.**

3. **As you exhale, bend forward from the waist and bring your head toward your knees and your hands forward and down toward the**

floor in the standing forward bend (see Figure 5-16c).

Keep your arms and legs soft (see Chapter 2 for an explanation of Forgiving Limbs). Pause.

4. **Bend your knees quite a bit and, as you inhale, sweep your arms out from the sides, but only come halfway up with your arms in a T (half forward bend), as shown in Figure 5-16d.**

Pause briefly.

5. **As you exhale, fold all the way down again and hang your arms in the standing forward bend (see Figure 5-16e).**

6. **As you inhale, sweep your arms from the sides like wings and bring your torso all the way up again, standing with your arms overhead in the standing arm raise (see Figure 5-16f).**

7. **As you exhale again, bring your arms back to your sides as in Step 1 (see Figure 5-16g).**

8. **Repeat the entire sequence six to eight times slowly.**

   On the last round, stay for six to eight breaths in the half forward bend (Step 4) and six to eight breaths in the standing forward bend (Step 5).

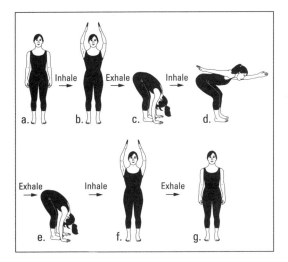

Figure 5-16: This series invigorates your entire torso, as well as your arms and legs.

Half chair

1. **Start in the mountain posture (refer to Figure 5-15). As you inhale, raise your arms forward, up and overhead, palms facing (see Figure 5-17a).**

2. **As you exhale, bend your knees and squat half-way to the floor.**

3. **Soften your arms but keep them overhead; look straight ahead (see Figure 5-17b).**

4. **Repeat Steps 1 through 3 three times, and then stay in the half chair posture (Step 3) for six to eight breaths.**

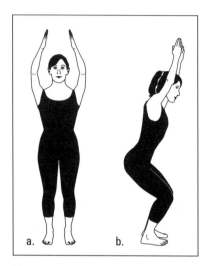

Figure 5-17: Anyone in favor of firm thighs?

Standing forward bend

Repeat the posture shown in Figure 5-7 in the "Beginner 1, Part I" section. Remain folded for six to eight breaths.

Balancing cat

1. **Begin on your hands and knees, place your hands directly under your shoulders, palms spread on the floor, with your knees directly under your hips.**

   Straighten your arms, but don't lock your elbows.

2. **As you exhale, slide your right hand forward and your left leg back, keeping your hand and toes on the floor.**

3. **As you inhale, raise your right arm and left leg as high as is comfortably possible for you (see Figure 5-18).**

   Stay for six to eight breaths.

4. **Repeat with opposite pairs (left arm and right leg).**

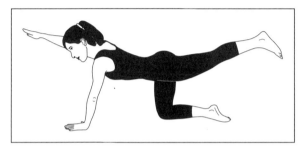

Figure 5-18: A classic posture for balancing the spinals, the small muscles in your back.

Corpse posture

Refer to Figure 5-1 in the "Beginner 1, Part I" section. Relax in this posture for eight to ten breaths.

Beginner 2, Part II

You're probably in week 7 of our eight-week program, and you're now reasonably competent in the exercises of Beginner 1 (Parts I and II) and Beginner 2 (Part I). Beginner 2, Part II, offers you more of a cardiovascular workout than Beginner 1. Don't be concerned if you find that you're perspiring when doing

these exercises. As your body cleans out from applying Yoga as a lifestyle, your perspiration becomes
odorless anyway.

Extended leg slide-ups

1. **Lie on your back, knees bent, feet flat on the
   floor at hip width.**

2. **Bend your left elbow and place your left hand
   on the back of your head, just behind your left
   ear.**

3. **Raise your left leg toward the vertical, but keep
   your knee slightly bent.**

   Draw the top of your foot toward the shin (to flex
   the ankle) and place your right palm on your
   right thigh near your pelvis (see Figure 5-19a).

4. **As you exhale, slowly sit up halfway and slide
   your right hand toward your knee.**

   Keep your left elbow back in line with your shoulder and look at the ceiling. Don't push your head
   forward (see Figure 5-19b).

5. **As you inhale, roll back slowly and return to
   Step 1.**

6. **Repeat Steps 4 and 5 six to eight times.**

7. **Repeat the same sequence on the opposite side.**

If this posture bothers your neck, support your
head with both hands behind your head. If the
problem persists, stop the exercise.

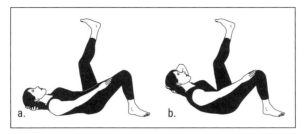

Figure 5-19: This posture works the abs and the hamstrings — a great combination!

Dynamic bridge

1. Lie on your back, knees bent, feet flat on the floor at hip width.

2. Place your arms at your sides, palms turned down (see Figure 5-20a).

3. As you inhale, raise your hips to a comfortable height (see Figure 5-20b).

4. As you exhale, return your hips to the floor.

5. Repeat Steps 3 and 4 six to eight times.

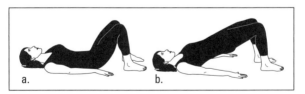

Figure 5-20: The bridge compensates or neutralizes the muscles you used in the slide-ups.

Locust 2

1. **Lie on your belly, and separate your legs to hip width, extend your toes, and lay the tops of your feet on the floor.**

   Place your forehead on the floor.

2. **Extend your right arm forward, palm resting on the floor; extend your left arm back behind you and let it rest on the floor near your left side, palm up (see Figure 5-21a).**

3. **As you inhale, slowly raise your chest, head, right arm, and left leg up and away from the floor, as high as you feel comfortable.**

   Try to keep your right arm and ear in alignment and your left foot as high as your right hand (see Figure 5-21b).

4. **As you exhale, slowly lower your right arm, chest, head, and left leg to the floor at the same time.**

5. **Repeat Steps 3 and 4 three times, and then hold in the up position (Step 3) for six to eight breaths.**

6. **Repeat with your left arm and right leg.**

Be careful of locust variations that lift just the legs, which increases chest pressure, heart rate, and tension in the neck. Definitely avoid these variations if you have heart problems or hypertension.

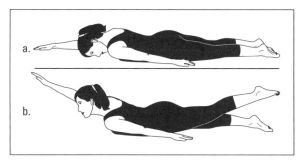

Figure 5-21: Try to bring the raised arm and foot to the same height.

Child's posture

Refer to Figure 5-5 in the "Beginner 1, Part I" section to perform this pose. Close your eyes and stay in the folded position for six to eight breaths.

Hamstring stretch

1. **Lie on your back, legs straight. Place your arms along your sides, palms down.**

2. **Bend your left knee and put your foot flat on the floor (refer to Figure 5-13a).**

3. **As you exhale, bring your right leg up as straight as possible (refer to Figure 5-13b).**

4. **As you inhale, return your leg to the floor.**

   Keep your head and the top of your hips on the floor.

5. **Repeat six to eight times, and then hold your leg up with your hands interlocked on the back of your raised thigh, just above the knee, for six to eight breaths (refer to Figure 5-13c).**

6. **Repeat Steps 1 through 5 with the legs reversed.**

Lift your head on a pillow or folded blanket if the back of your neck or your throat tenses when you raise or lower your leg.

Be very careful of all seated forward bends if you have disc-related back problems. Avoid these movements completely if you have pain or numbness in the back, buttocks, or legs.

Seated forward bend

1. **Sit on the floor with your legs at hip width and comfortably stretched out in front of you.**

   Bring your back up nice and tall and place your palms down on the floor near your thighs.

2. **As you inhale, raise your arms forward and up overhead until they're beside your ears.**

   Keep your arms and legs soft and slightly bent in Forgiving Limbs, as discussed in Chapter 2 (see Figure 5-22a).

3. **As you exhale, bend forward from the hips and bring your hands, chest, and head toward your legs.**

   Rest your hands on your thighs, knees, shins, or feet. If your head isn't close to your knees, bend your knees more until you feel your back stretching (see Figure 5-22b).

4. **Repeat Steps 2 and 3 three to four times, and then stay folded for six to eight breaths.**

If you have a problem sitting upright on the floor in the seated forward bend or any of the following forward-bending postures, raise your hips on a folded blanket or firm pillow (see Figure 5-22c).

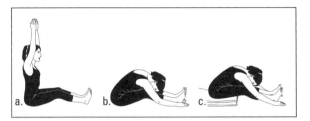

Figure 5-22: Forward bends are calming and quieting and often used toward the end of a routine.

Corpse posture

 To perform the corpse posture, refer to Figure 5-1 in the "Beginner 1, Part I" section. Relax in this posture for 15 to 30 breaths.

Chapter 6

Designing Your Own Yoga Program

- -

In This Chapter

▶ Introducing the classic formula

▶ Outlining 30- to 60-minute routines

▶ Presenting 15-minute routines

▶ Refreshing with a 5-minute routine

- -

*I*f you're like most people, you can't wait to cook up your own exercise routines. Opinions are plentiful about how to create an efficient Hatha Yoga program. In this chapter, we give you some practical guidelines, including a classic formula, that you can use to put together a variety of routines — exercises for different occasions throughout your life.

We don't intend for our advice to be a universal remedy. Some situations call for highly personalized attention. We're not offering a panacea for readers with serious muscular or skeletal problems, such as acute back pain, or those who have a serious illness. Providing a formula that fits every conceivable ailment or special circumstance is beyond the scope of this book — or any book.

If you're dealing with a specific health challenge, you need to work one on one, under the guidance of your doctor, with a Yoga therapist or other health professional. This chapter focuses on "do-it-yourself" Hatha Yoga for general conditioning and stress reduction. Our emphasis is on prevention rather than therapy.

In Chapter 5, we describe step-by-step procedures for using the main postures.

Cooking Up a Creative Course of Exercise with the Classic Formula

Creating your own Yoga program is not unlike figuring out how to create your own fabulous meals. You determine how much time you have and which cuisine you're likely to enjoy the most. You consult your cookbook about the principles of combining main and side dishes and preparing each one properly. When the food is cooked, you sit down and relish each bite. You eat slowly to savor every single morsel. When you finish, you don't jump up right away; instead, you sit back and relax for a while and let your stomach begin its digestive work.

When you create your own Yoga program with our classic formula, you

- ✔ Determine how long you want the routine to be.

- ✔ Select the main postures from the range of postures covered in Chapter 5 (or, of course, from any source you consider reliable).

- ✔ Decide how you want to prepare and/or compensate for each main category of postures.

- ✔ Allocate time for rest and relaxation at the end in order to digest the nutritious meal of Yoga exercises that you prepared for yourself.

What we call the Classic Formula consists of the following 12 categories:

1. **Attunement (integrating body, mind, and breath)**
2. **Preparation or warm-up (also used between main exercises wherever necessary)**
3. **Standing postures**
4. **Balance postures (optional)**
5. **Abdominals**
6. **Inversions (optional)**
7. **Back bends**
8. **Forward bends**
9. **Twists**
10. **Rest (to be inserted between main exercises whenever you feel the need)**
11. **Compensation (to be inserted after main exercises)**
12. **Final relaxation**

You don't have to use all these categories as long as you follow the proper sequence (from 1 to 9 and always concluding with 12). The categories of *rest, preparation/warm-up,* and *compensation* are repeated where appropriate. Balancing postures, and inversions are marked *optional,* because their inclusion depends on your available time.

The Classic Formula is optimal for 30- to 60-minute general conditioning programs, but we also refer to it in the 15- and 5-minute programs. The beauty of our formula is that, as your Yoga practice grows over the years, you can explore safe postures from any book or system and then insert them into their appropriate slots within our 12-category module.

Enjoying a Postural Feast: The 30- to 60-Minute General Conditioning Routine

An old saying proposes that you can give someone a fish or you can hand that person a fishing pole and teach him how to fish. In a similar way, we can just offer you some precooked Yoga routines as we do in Chapter 5, or we can teach you how to cook up your own postural feasts.

Most beginning Yoga students find it difficult to sustain more than a 30- minute practice on their own; however, if your appetite increases, we want you to have the tools to be a 60-minute gourmet. Simply follow the recipes in each of the categories to create your own great, custom routine.

If you live 70 years, you spend 23 years asleep and about 6 years preparing meals and eating. If you watch only one hour of television a day (and most people watch a lot more), this adds up to an amazing three years in your lifetime. How much time do we spend shopping, commuting, reading advertisements, and so on? Scary, isn't it? In light of this, even 30 to 60 minutes of Yoga practice five times a week seems more than reasonable, especially considering that Yoga may well extend your life span.

An average of about two minutes for each posture you select is a good general yardstick for planning your practice time. Some postures take more time, some take less. An asymmetrical or

two-sided (right and left) posture like the warrior is counted as one exercise or posture. If you
choose a sun salutation or a similar dynamic
series from another source, double or triple the
time allotted, depending on the series and the
number of rounds.

Note: Many of these postures are versatile: You can
often use some of the same postures in more than
one category when developing a general conditioning
routine.

Attunement

To help you understand *attunement* — your personal
connectedness — think of it this way: Attunement is
like logging on to the Internet. Your "password" is the
type of breathing you select for your attunement and
the rest of your program. After you log on and estab-
lish the conscious link between your body, breath,
and mind, all the benefits of the Yoga universe are
yours. If you forget about the attunement stage, you'll
be logged off the cosmic Internet before you have a
chance to receive all the benefits of your Hatha Yoga
session.

First, for routines of any length, select a style of
breathing from Chapter 4. If you're a beginner, choose
something simple like focus breathing or belly
breathing.

Next, select a resting posture or a sitting posture,
depending on your frame of mind, your physical con-
dition, or what you have planned for the rest of your
routine. The corpse posture (lying flat on your back)
is always a good starting point for beginners. With

our hectic lifestyles, we usually need to shift gears and slow things down before we can begin our postural exercises. Lying flat on your back definitely shifts your mood toward relaxation. However, sitting in the easy posture or standing in the mountain posture also makes a great starting point. Figure 6-1 shows some examples of rest postures that you can use to help achieve attunement.

Use 8 to 12 breaths to achieve attunement. The more you "remember" (pay attention to) the breath and your attunement, the more benefit you can expect to derive from your program.

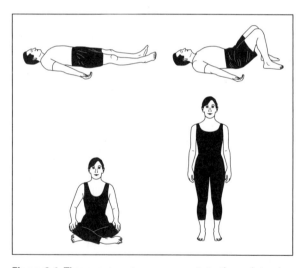

Figure 6-1: These rest postures are great starting points when working toward attunement.

Warm-up

You may notice that almost all Yoga warm-ups are folding and opening motions (flexion and extension). Either motion provides the easiest way for your body to prepare for breath and movement. Select a warm-up posture or sequence that is a *similar* position to your attunement posture.

 Make your Yoga practice as smooth as possible. Flow like a gentle river. For example, your attunement and warm-up both can take place on the floor; then you can stand up for all the standing postures. Avoid getting up and down like a yo-yo. Economy of movement is one of the principles of good Hatha Yoga practice.

 If you're composing a routine designed for 30 minutes or more, you usually have room for at least two warm-up postures. Because the neck is a frequent site of tension, we often suggest using a warm-up posture that incorporates moving the arms. In addition to stretching the spine, arm movement prepares your neck and shoulders and helps you release tension. Also, warm-ups that move the legs and prepare the lower back are helpful for the standing postures that usually follow.

Check out Figure 6-2 for some examples of common warm-ups in the lying, sitting, and standing positions.

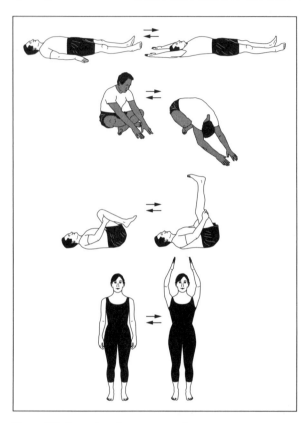

Figure 6-2: Examples of warm-up postures.

Standing postures

The standing postures tend to be the most "physical"
part of a program. If you're doing a 30-minute routine,

you usually have time for three or four standing postures. In a 60-minute program, you may have as many as six or seven main *asanas*. You can choose any of the standing postures for this portion of your routine.

Before you begin picking your postures, run through a simple rule of sequencing: Back bends, twists, and side bends are usually followed by forward bends. Therefore, you want to include standing forward bends after most of the standing postures you choose.

Figure 6-3 shows you examples of standing postures for a 30-minute or 60-minute program. As an alternative, you can also choose the dynamic kneeling or standing sequence (sun salutation) or the standing rejuvenation sequence for beginners from Chapter 5.

In terms of time, the dynamic postures take the place of three to six standing postures, depending on which sequence you choose and how many rounds you do. When you select a dynamic sequence, try to allow time at the end for one twist and one compensating forward bend. We mention this because all our dynamic sequences are forward and backward bends only.

 If you want your routine to be more physically challenging, simply do two sets of the standing postures.

 The simplest way to expand a 30-minute routine into a 45-minute routine is to do two sets of your chosen standing postures and add one extra posture to the abdominal, back bend, and forward bend categories.

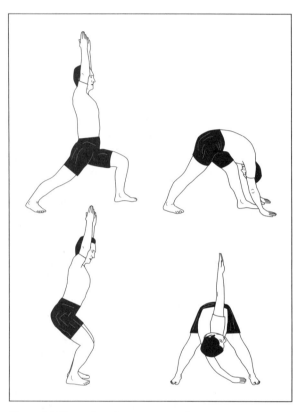

Figure 6-3: Examples of common standing postures.

Balancing postures (optional)

Balancing postures are optional and depend on your time and stamina. They're often the most athletic postures and require overall coordination. Balancing postures are very rewarding, because you can see your progress immediately. They fit nicely after the standing postures because at this point in your routine, you're fully warmed up. Also, all our recommended balancing postures are either standing or kneeling, which means they fit smoothly into the sequence. Choose one balancing posture (see Figure 6-4) for a 30-minute to 60-minute routine.

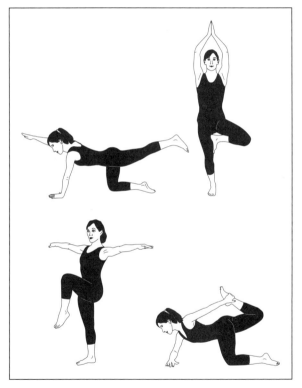

Figure 6-4: Examples of balancing postures.

Rest

Most people usually welcome a rest at this point, and rest works nicely after any strenuous portion of your routine. Resting is usually done lying, sitting, or kneeling. We emphasize the importance of not feeling rushed during your Yoga session. At least for the short duration of your routine, believe that you have all the time in the world. In a 30- or 60-minute routine, the first rest usually comes at the halfway point. This resting period gives you the opportunity for inward observation of any physical, mental, or emotional feedback resulting from your Yoga practice so far.

You need to rest until you feel ready to move on. If you're really pinched for time, this first major rest is also a logical place to stop a session. Select a posture from Figure 6-1.

Abdominals

The belly is a focal point for exercise-conscious Americans. We recommend that you include at least one, but not more than two, abdominal postures in any program lasting 30 minutes or more. Think of your abdomen as "the front of your back" — a very important place. Choose one abdominal posture (see Figure 6-5) for a 30-minute routine or one or two for a 60-minute routine.

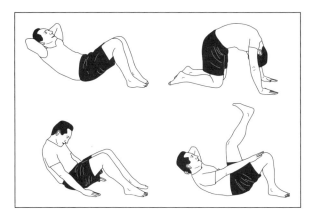

Figure 6-5: Abdominal postures strengthen the front of your back.

Compensation and preparation

Take a short rest when you finish the abdominal exercises and then use the dynamic bridge, the dynamic bridge with arm variation, or the lying arm raise six to eight times (see Figure 6-6). The action of the dynamic bridge plays a dual function here, because it *compensates* the abdomen, returning it to neutral. The bridge also warms up or *prepares* the back and the neck, if you choose to include an inversion posture or move on to back bends next.

Note: Compensation and preparation are normally done dynamically (moving).

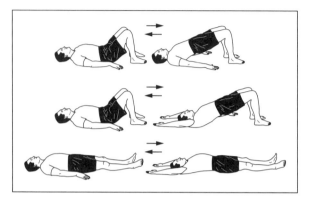

Figure 6-6: Compensation for abdominals can also be preparation for inversions.

Inversion (optional)

Indian Yoga teachers often teach inverted postures toward the beginning or at the end of a class. For Westerners, we prefer inverted postures closer to the middle of the program, when they've properly prepared their backs and necks and they have plenty of time for adequate compensation. Inverted postures, like those shown in Figure 6-7, are optional, and we recommend that beginners avoid the half shoulder stand and the half shoulder stand at the wall until they've practiced Yoga for six to eight weeks.

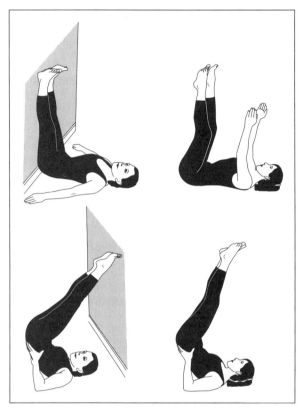

Figure 6-7: Inversions are powerful postures that deserve respect.

Even after you're comfortable with your yogic practice, attempt inversions only if you have no neck problems. Inverted postures are worthy of a healthy respect rather than fear. They're powerful postures, but they demand a sense of balance and strong muscles. Select just one inversion posture for your 30- to 60- minute routine, assuming you're ready and you want to include an inversion in your practice.

We advise against practicing the half shoulder stand or the half shoulder stand at the wall if:

- ✔ You have glaucoma.

- ✔ You have high blood pressure.

- ✔ You have a history of heart attacks or stroke.

- ✔ You have a hiatal hernia.

- ✔ You're in the first few days of menstruation.

- ✔ You're pregnant.

- ✔ You're currently 40 or more pounds overweight.

Compensation for inversions and preparation for back bends

You should rest after the simpler inverted postures, normally in the corpse posture. After the half shoulder stand, rest and then compensate further with any one of the cobra postures or the thunderbolt posture. The cobra and thunderbolt posture also prepare you for further back bends. Figure 6-8 shows these examples.

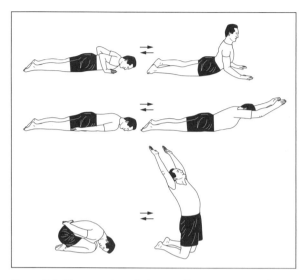

Figure 6-8: These postures help you either compensate for an inversion or prepare for deeper back bends.

Back bends

Check for yourself how well back bends work after an inverted posture, and also how the cobra is an excellent compensation for the shoulder stand. The cobra also is a gentle back bend that serves as good preparation for more physical back bends, such as the locust posture.

As Westerners, we bend forward far too much — that fact makes back bends a vital part of your Hatha Yoga practice. Whenever possible in general conditioning

Yoga routines, select one back bend; in programs over 30 minutes, select two back bends. Figure 6-9 shows some common back bends you can try.

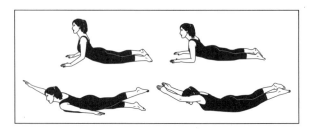

Figure 6-9: Examples of four common back bends.

Compensation for back bends

The compensation for prone back bends is usually some form of a bent knee forward bend (see Figure 6-10). We often recommend the knees-to-chest or the child's posture. After more strenuous back bends, such as any of the varieties of the locust postures, we suggest a short rest, followed by one of the bent knee forward bends, and then the dynamic bridge posture as a second compensatory posture. This sequence helps neutralize the upper back and neck.

Preparation for forward bends

Preparation is particularly critical in the performance of extended leg forward bends. Stretching the hamstrings or the hips just before any of the recommended seated forward bends not only improves the posture but also is safer for your back. Use the hamstring stretch, or the double leg stretch for a 30-minute routine. For a longer routine, use both and/or the rock-the-baby sequence (see Figure 6-11).

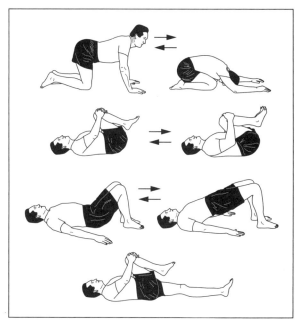

Figure 6-10: Compensating for back bends is an important part of your Yoga program.

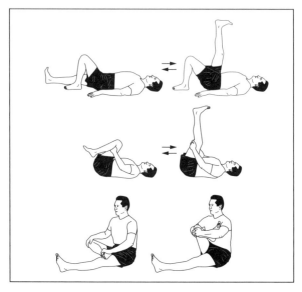

Figure 6-11: These postures help you prepare for forward bends.

Forward bends

The seated forward bends are normally done toward the end of an exercise program because they have a calming effect. Of all the postures described in this book, the seated extended leg forward bends divide the sexes the most. Men have a higher muscle density, especially in the hip and groin area and are usually tighter in the hamstrings. Preparation of the hamstrings is particularly important. If you have a hard time with this category, bend your knees more and, if necessary, place some blankets under your hips to give yourself a better angle for the forward bends.

For a 30-minute routine, choose just one forward
bend. For a 60-minute routine, select two forward
bends (see Figure 6-12).

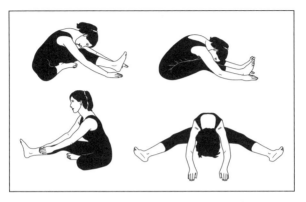

Figure 6-12: Examples of forward bends.

Compensation for forward bends

The forward bends are usually self-compensating.
However, sometimes you may want to use a gentle
back bend like the dynamic bridge as a counter pose.

Preparation for twists

The preparation for all twists is a forward bend. So,
moving from the category of forward bends to twists
is another grouping in the classic schema that flows
naturally.

Twists

Twists, like forward bends, have an overall calming effect. The floor twists are the dessert in our program, because at the end of the routine they just feel so good. Choose one floor twist for a 30-minute routine and one or two floor twists for a 60-minute routine. Figure 6-13 shows some common twists.

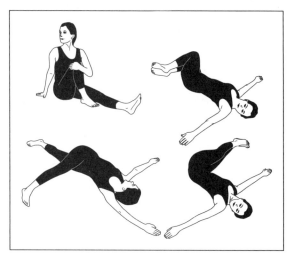

Figure 6-13: Twists are calming postures, and they just feel good.

Compensation for twists

Compensation for twists is always flexion, or a forward bend. After a floor twist, we usually recommend choosing one of the lying knees-to-chest or the knee-to-chest posture (see Figure 6-14).

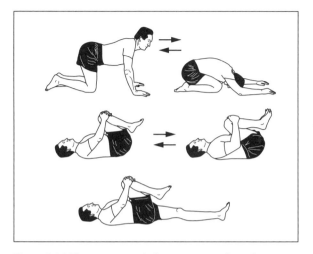

Figure 6-14: These postures help compensate for twists.

Relaxation

No matter how short your program, remember to include some form of relaxation. Rest provides a place where "absorption" can take place: You digest all the marvelous energies unleashed by your Yoga exercises.

This final category in our classic formula can take several forms: a relaxation technique, yogic breathing called *pranayama* (see Chapter 4), or meditation.

First, choose one of the rest postures or one of the sitting postures. Next, select one of the breathing or *pranayama* techniques from Chapter 4, a relaxation technique from Chapter 3, and/or a meditation technique. In a 60-minute routine, you may choose both a breathing and a relaxation technique.

Whichever technique you choose, use it for at least 2 to 3 minutes and not more than 15 minutes.

Making the Most of Little: A 15-Minute Routine

Face it, available time is often limited. But rather than shelve your Yoga practice (and well-being), you can settle happily for a mini-routine. Even 15 minutes of Hatha Yoga can put you back on an even keel or remind your body and mind of how good stretching, moving, and breathing feel.

If we're honest with ourselves, most of us tend to spend a fair amount of time in idle motion — not really resting but not working either. Just picture revving your car engine when you're parked. We all have at least 15 minutes every day that we can put to good use to fortify our physical and mental health and/or put a dollar into our spiritual savings account.

When you opt for a 15-minute program, you need to be specific about your goals. Some of the more common uses for a short routine are

- ✔ A quick general conditioning program
- ✔ A stress-reduction and relaxation program
- ✔ A preparation program for Yoga breathing or meditation

General conditioning

For the purposes of general conditioning, choose the following categories and do them in the order listed.

You can also use the illustrations earlier in this chapter as a reference point.

- ✔ Either a standing or sitting rest posture for attunement (refer to Figure 16-1) and a Yoga breathing technique from Chapter 4

- ✔ A dynamic series, such as either kneeling or standing sun salutation; the rejuvenation sequence, which counts as three or four postures (see Chapter 5); or three to four standing postures (refer to Figure 6-3) for six to eight minutes

- ✔ A lying twist (refer to Figure 6-13)

- ✔ Compensate with knees or knee-to-chest postures (refer to Figure 6-14)

- ✔ A lying or sitting rest posture (refer to Figure 6-1)

- ✔ A breathing exercise (see Chapter 4) and/or a relaxation technique (see Chapter 3)

Preparation for meditation and Yoga breathing

If you're looking for a routine to help you reduce stress, just plain relax, or prepare for meditation and Yoga breathing, choose the following elements, and do them in the order listed:

- ✔ A lying or sitting posture for attunement (refer to Figure 6-1) and a Yoga breathing technique from Chapter 4

- ✔ Two lying warm-up postures, one that moves the arms and the other that moves the legs (refer to Figure 6-2)

✔ A *supine* (lying on your belly) back-bending posture such as the cobra or locust (refer to Figure 6-9) or a lying back bend such as the bridge (refer to Figure 6-6)

✔ A bent knee compensation exercise such as the child's pose or knees to chest (refer to Figure 6-10)

✔ A lying hamstring posture (refer to Figure 6-11)

✔ A lying twist (refer to Figure 6-13)

✔ A lying bent knee compensation exercise (refer to Figure 6-14)

✔ A lying or sitting rest posture (refer to Figure 6-1) with a breathing exercise (see Chapter 4) and/or a relaxation technique (see Chapter 3)

Satisfying an Appetite for a Quick Pick-Me-Up: A Five-Minute Routine

A five-minute program is the easiest to create. For a busy person, even three to five minutes once or twice a day can provide beneficial effects. Choose a rest posture or a sitting posture from Figure 6-1 and then select a yogic breathing or *pranayama* technique (see Chapter 4) for three to five minutes. You'll not only enjoy a quick, relaxing routine, but you'll also have at least 60 possible combinations to choose from.

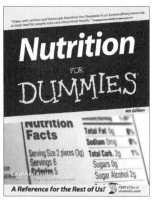
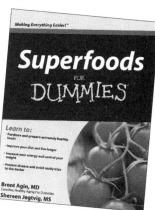
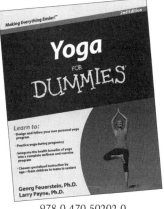
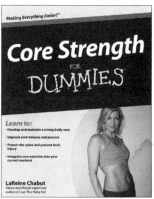

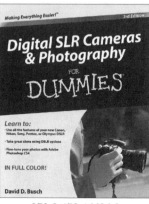
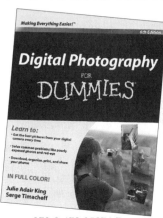
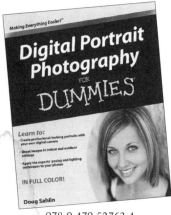
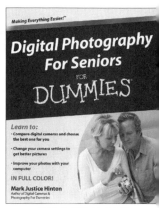

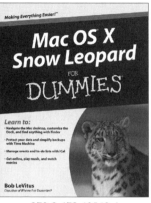
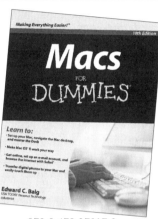
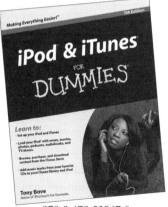
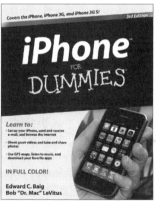

After you've read the Portable Edition, look for the original Dummies book on the topic. The handy Contents at a Glance below highlights the information you'll get when you purchase a copy of *Yoga For Dummies* — available wherever books are sold, or visit dummies.com.

Contents at a Glance